BOERHAAVE SERIES
FOR POSTGRADUATE
MEDICAL EDUCATION
Vol. 14

PROCEEDINGS OF BOERHAAVE COURSES
ORGANIZED BY
THE FACULTY OF MEDICINE, UNIVERSITY OF LEIDEN,
THE NETHERLANDS

THERAPEUTIC RELEVANCE OF DRUG ASSAYS

THERAPEUTIC RELEVANCE OF DRUG ASSAYS

edited by

F.A. DE WOLFF, Ph.D., M.D., H. MATTIE, M.D.
Leiden University Hospital
and
D.D. BREIMER, Ph.D.
Department of Pharmacology, Leiden University

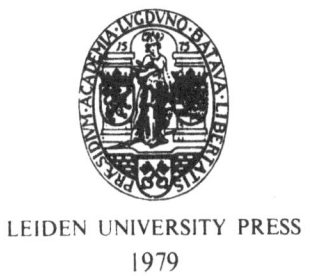

LEIDEN UNIVERSITY PRESS
1979

The distribution of this book is handled by the following team of publishers:

for the United States and Canada

Kluwer Boston, Inc.
160 Old Derby Street
Hingham, MA 02043
USA

for all other countries

Kluwer Academic Publishers Group
Distribution Center
P.O. Box 322
3300 AH Dordrecht
The Netherlands

Library of Congress Cataloging in Publication Data   CIP

Main entry under title:

Therapeutic relevance of drug assays.

  (Boerhaave series for postgraduate medical education; v. 14)
  Includes bibliographies and index.
  1. Drugs – Analysis. 2. Body fluids – Analysis. 3. Chemotherapy. I. Wolff, F.A.
de. II. Mattie, H. III. Breimer, Douwe D., 1943–   IV. Series.
[DNLM: 1. Drug evaluation – Congresses. 2. Drug industry – Congresses. 3. Drugs –
Standards – Congresses.
W3 B0672 no. 14/QV771 T398]
RS189.T44   615′.7   79–15103

ISBN-13:978-94-009-9585-7   e-ISBN-13:978-94-009-9583-3
DOI: 10.1007/978-94-009-9583-3

Cover design: Paul Burg

Copyright © 1979 by Martinus Nijhoff Publishers bv, The Hague/Boston/London.
Softcover reprint of the hardcover 1st edition 1979

FOREWORD

The desirability of quality-assay of ingestable or imbibable material has resulted in an established procedure in advanced countries. Testimony to its necessity was borne by the scandal of chateau-bottled Bordeaux *crus classés* a few years ago, a litigation instigated by the disillusioned consumers who either on the basis of absence of the expected inebriate state, or of the olfacto-gustatory caress by the bouquet or full-bodied lingering pharyngeal sensation, decided to strike a paranoid attitude, which ultimately proved to be justified.

When one proceeds from sheer pleasure to dire necessity, the question of what happens to ingested medication assumes quite portentous features. Testimony is borne to this by the transitional stage, at which one is faced with the legal consequences of the basically illegal alcohol-respiration test, based on the relationship between the amount of ingested alcohol and the C_2H_5OH concentration in expired air or in venous blood, a wholly unconstitutional terror, in view of the Rome treaty signed by the Western countries, which says that nobody should be required to cooperate in procedures aimed at providing him guilty. On top of this, the lamentable fact is observable, that among the *professio nobile* there are even those who took the oath of Hippocrates and lend their hands, not to cure (as they promised), but to perform a cubital vein puncture in order to prove someone, who is not their patient, guilty.

The fate of medically active substances within a compartmentalized organism is being unravelled, mainly in the clinical toxicology and pharmacology departments, a laudable, meritorious and necessary effort. Recent years have witnessed such a mushrooming development in this field that today, in many hospitals, in both the emergency wards and outpatient departments of internal medicine, cardiology, neurology, and psychiatry, therapeutic management of the patient would be like a blind date if one did not have the monitoring of intravital drug levels at one's hands.

This book, based on a Boerhaave course on the essence and impact of drug assays, designed and crystallized by our clinical pharmacophilic trio Drs. de Wolff, Mattie, and Breimer, should convince those reading it that therapeutic drug assay does indeed strike a harmonious theme, potentially rich in variations, fully in concert with the ultimate goals of the *dramatis personae*, the patient, physician, and pharmacologist, in question. Pitfalls, such as physicians' incompetence, patient's non-compliance, and pharmaceutic inefficacy, will be discordantly revealed if the play truly follows its plot.

As a rather old-fashioned doctor, I feel for honesty's sake that I should not keep you unaware of my reserves *vis à vis* any judgement on drug treatment of a patient. This critical attitude was instilled by one of my teachers who, during his ward rounds, used to remark to any suggestion of drug therapy for a patient: "Another colour shoeshine will help him as well." This sophisticated disdain of the pseudo-magic act of prescribing a drug (And who among us do not know from experience many a bitter disappointment?) was translated into a playful persiflage by a recent writer in a deceased journal of which I was one of the editors.

This writer reported the qualities of a panacea called Nietsch®. Its pharmacokinetics adapted themselves miraculously to the species of animals to which it was being experimentally administered prior to clinical trial (fig. 1). Its conversion to ethanol and its other remarkable properties resulting from elimination of N- or Ch-radicals were proposed in dramatic fashion in the *Journal of Phony Results* (fig. 2), an unjustifiably ill-read journal which essentially is a condensation of all articles usually published in pharmaceutic and medical journals. The drug was withdrawn from the market for reasons obscure. An intimation of them however is provided by the curve of the drug's maximal dose effect (fig. 3), which clearly proves that the pharmaceutic

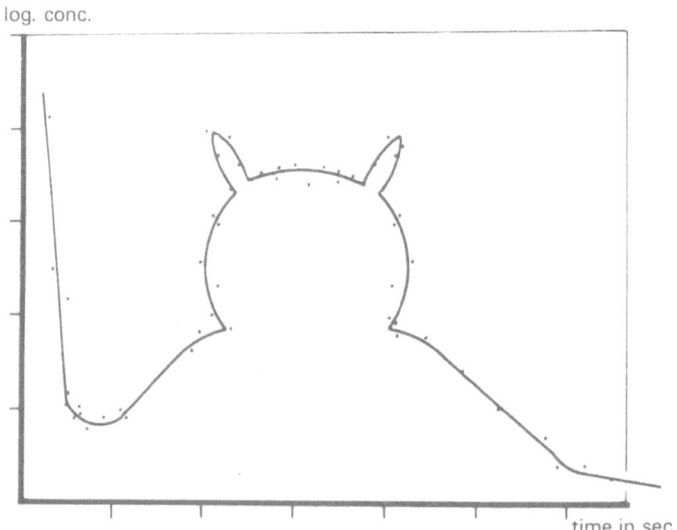

Figure 1. Pharmacokinetics of Nietsch® revealed by experimental administration prior to clinical trial.

competitors must have bought the formula in panic and destroyed it: "Quid rides? Mutato nomine de te fabula narratur!" (Horatius *Saturn* 1, 1, 69).

The experienced physician subscribes to the rationalization (i.e. quantification, reasoning, and logic regulation) of therapeutic measures, allowing

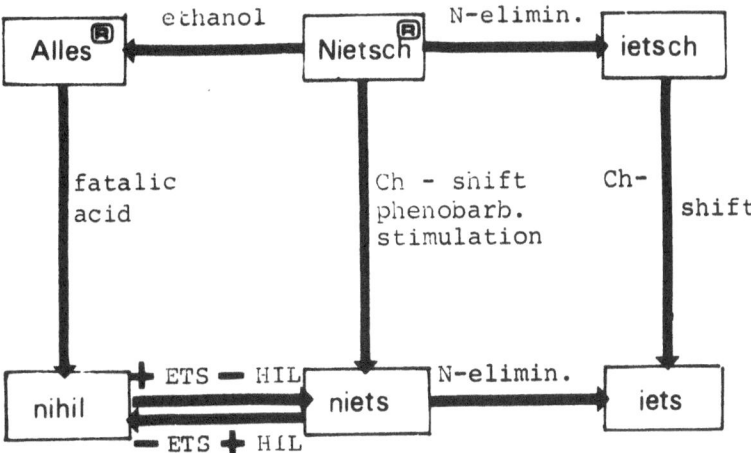

Figure 2. Conversion of Nietsch[®] to ethanol and its properties resulting from elimination of N- or Ch-radicals. (H.A. Godomski, Pharmacokinetics of the MODEL. *Journal of Phony Results* 1, 1-100, 1978.)

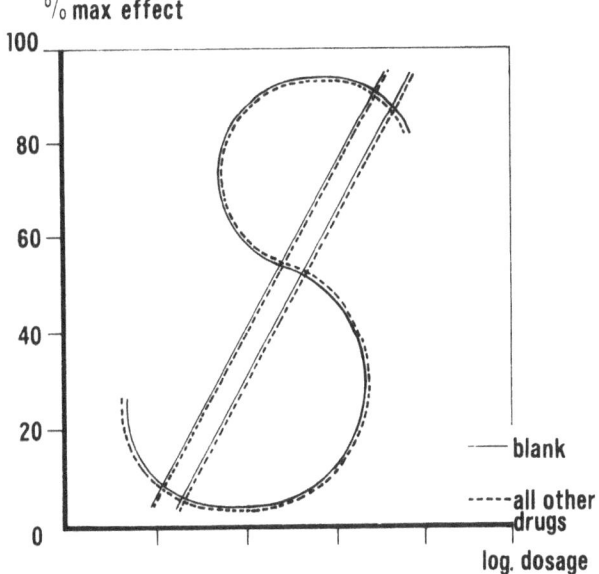

Figure 3. Maximal dose effect of the drug Nietsch.[®]

for the imponderable factors in the process of cure as yet untouched by the light of scientific progress.

As such, this book is aimed at contributing to augment the rational control of the action of drugs in diseased man. If it materially succeeds in showing today's inapplicability of Voltaire's dictum: "Un médecin est un homme, qui met des drogues, qu'il ne connaît pas, dans un corps, qu'il connaît encore moins," this volume will be a successful one, and its editors will be fully rewarded.

G.W. BRUYN

CONTENTS

CONTRIBUTORS

A. AMDISEN, Psychopharmacology Research Unit, Psychiatric Hospital of Aarhus, Risskov, Denmark.

A.M. BRECKENRIDGE, Department of Pharmacology and Therapeutics, University Hospital, Liverpool, United Kingdom.

D.D. BREIMER, Department of Pharmacology, Subfaculty of Pharmacy, State University, Leiden, The Netherlands.

G.W. BRUYN, Department of Neurology, University Hospital, Leiden, The Netherlands.

A.N.P. VAN HEIJST, Department of Reanimation and Clinical Toxicology, University Hospital, Utrecht, The Netherlands.

E. VAN DER KLEIJN, Department of Clinical Pharmacy, St. Radboud Hospital, Catholic University, Nijmegen, The Netherlands.

P. KRAGH-SØRENSEN, Department of Psychiatry, University Hospital, Odense, Denmark.

H. MATTIE, Department of Clinical Pharmacology, University Hospital, Leiden, The Netherlands.

G.E. MAWER, Department of Pharmacology, Materia Medica and Therapeutics, University of Manchester, Manchester, United Kingdom.

E.L. NOACH, Department of Pharmacology, Faculty of Medicine, State University, Leiden, The Netherlands.

L. OFFERHAUS, Department of Pharmacotherapy, Ministry of Public Health and Environmental Hygiene, Leidschendam, The Netherlands.

M.L'E. ORME, Department of Pharmacology and Therapeutics, University Hospital, Liverpool, United Kingdom.

H.M. PINEDO, University Hospital, Netherlands Cancer Institute and Department of Oncology, Free University, Amsterdam, The Netherlands.

A. RICHENS, Department of Clinical Pharmacology, St. Bartholomew's Hospital, London, United Kingdom.

H. TIMMERS, Department of Internal Medicine, Wilhelmina Gasthuis, Amsterdam, The Netherlands.

T.B. VREE, Department of Clinical Pharmacy, St. Radboud Hospital, Catholic University, Nijmegen, The Netherlands.

H. WESSELING, Institute for Clinical Pharmacology, University of Groningen, Groningen, The Netherlands.

B. WIDDOP, Poisons Unit, New Cross Hospital, London, United Kingdon.

P.M. WILKINSON, Christie Hospital and Holt Radium Institute, Withington, Manchester, United Kingdom.

F.A. DE WOLFF, Laboratory of Toxicology, University Hospital, Leiden, The Netherlands.

PART I

GENERAL ASPECTS

1. THERAPEUTIC RELEVANCE OF DRUG ASSAYS

H. MATTIE

There are several reasons why quantities of drugs in body fluids of patients should be determined. Some of these have to do with the individual patient's benefit, some with the advancement of medicine, and of course often both goals are aimed at. Apart from this, the possibility of estimating serum and urinary concentrations of drugs in experiments on healthy volunteers has led to a much better understanding of the biological properties of the pharmaceutic formulation of a drug: whether oral administration is as effective as parenteral administration, what properties good tablets or good suppositories should have, and so on. In this chapter we will limit ourselves to the question of why a doctor should ask for the determination of drugs in a patient.

ESTABLISHING DIAGNOSIS OF DISEASE

First of all, the determination of the presence of drugs in a patient may be a diagnostic procedure. Drugs nowadays are not a rare cause of disease, whether or not they are applied skilfully. Because side effects of drugs are not always exaggerations of the intended therapeutic effect, it is not always unequivocally clear whether a patient has acquired a second disease, or whether he is suffering from the treatment of the initial disease. Even when the side effect is explainable by the drug it is not always dependent upon dose or concentration. This may be explained by some examples. When somebody is drunk, it is assumed that he has had too much alcohol. The diagnosis is often made by observation and common sense on the basis of a few characteristic signs: behaviour and smell, and a history of alcohol consumption. That will suffice in most instances. Nevertheless, even without the possibility of determining alcohol concentrations in blood, it has always been well known that some people can stand much larger quantities of alcohol than others, most often because of adaptation of the central nervous system. Therefore, the question may be asked why alcohol concentrations should be determined when it is known beforehand that a concentration of 1.5 g/l may be consistent with apparently normal behaviour in some people, while a concentration of 0.5 g/l leads to patently abnormal behaviour in others. There are many other examples of diagnostic signs that are equivocal in the same way: a normal temperature in a patient who is in shock does not exclude severe infection; a normal serum bilirubin does not exclude an obstruction of the biliary duct, at least when it is recent. However, this has never led to abandoning this kind of test altogether. The point to be made is that doctors have learned to work with this kind of data and that they also have to learn the relative importance of serum concentrations of drugs, together with other signs and symptoms, to establish a diagnosis. In the present example: a low alcohol concentration in an experienced drinker, together with grossly abnormal behaviour, will lead to a careful neurological examination, because there might be a serious cerebral lesion. The history alone is insufficient in those cases, because of its known unreliability in heavy drinkers.

GATHERING KNOWLEDGE OF DISEASE

A second good reason for the drug determination is that apart from the useful information obtained from individual patients it may have wider implications. For instance, if alcohol concentrations had not been determined in many otherwise healthy people, or in patients with neurological or endocrine disorders, or in habitual heavy drinkers, we would not have known some important facts, for instance, the fact that habituation to the toxic effect of alcohol in alcoholists is not the result of more rapid metabolism in the liver; or, that acute hepatitis in an alcoholic should not be diagnosed as alcohol hepatitis when there is no alcohol present. Therefore, whenever a doctor thinks of asking for a drug determination, he should ask himself whether he needs it to establish a diagnosis, or to obtain a better insight into the disease in general, as is, or should be, with all diagnostic procedures. The latter indication, the advancement of the knowledge of the disease, is often overlooked. This leads to the erroneous conclusion that if a determination cannot be done immediately it should not be done at all. It may indeed be useless for the patient himself, but the same can be said of an autopsy, and probably nobody will deny the importance of the consistent verification of a diagnosis by pathologic examination. There is, however, a problem that makes drug determinations different from other diagnostic procedures, being that many doctors have not learned to interpret this kind of laboratory finding. For a proper interpretation of a certain drug concentration it is necessary to have some knowledge of the relation between concentration and effect, and of the time relations between administration, concentration and effect. Again this may be illustrated by an example concerning alcohol. The Dutch law allows not more than 0.5 g/1 (50 mg/100 ml) of alcohol in the blood for driving. That is not because this is an absolutely safe level, but because of the above-mentioned relations. When blood alcohol is determined some time after an accident, in most instances the actual level at the time of the accident will have been higher, but how much higher is not easy to tell. It is however possible to make a more accurate guess, by a second determination, some time later, so that the amount of alcohol metabolism in the individual subject may be determined by the difference of the two determinations. The exception is, of course, when the accident took place a very short time after the alcohol ingestion. In this case the alcohol percentage at the time of the test may be *higher* than at the time of the accident, because alcohol was still being absorbed. This does not really excuse the driver, because the mental instability is probably greater with a rapidly rising alcohol level, than with a slowly declining one. This example may illustrate that the maximal diagnostic information can be derived from a drug determination only when all clinical, pharmacological and technical aspects are considered.

Drugs as the cause of disease
In this respect something more should be said about drugs as causes of disease. Some adverse reactions to drugs are more likely to be concentration-dependent than others. When the unwanted effect is an exaggerated pharmacological one it is often concentration-dependent: e.g., extreme sedation by sedatives, deafness by aspirin, bone marrow depression by chloramphenicol. It should be noticed that these are not only exaggerations of the *intended* therapeutic effect, but also well-known pharmacological effects that are unrelated to it. In those instances a drug determination can sometimes establish or confirm the diagnosis or exclude it. Even so the individual sensitivity to a drug at a certain concentration level may vary widely. Sometimes this is firmly established quantitatively, but most often only uncontrolled clinical experience gives us some knowledge of the variation in drug response between individuals. To form this clinical experience it is indeed necessary to collect enough data on the correlation between concentration and effect. In clinical practice every doctor has to decide for himself whether he will rely wholly on data from the literature, or whether he deems it necessary to form his own experience. In this respect it should be mentioned that unfortunately much literature data on the relation between concentration and therapeutic or toxic effect is not so much established facts as opinion.

In general, some toxic effects, for instance those on liver or kidney, tend to be rather closely related to concentration, and more so than many therapeutic effects. One might speculate that this is so, because the therapeutic effects depend a great deal on the state of the disease, which is in itself very variable. Therefore, to avoid toxic concentrations a drug assay is often indicated. A whole class of adverse reactions is not concentration-related, namely the allergic manifestations. Measurement of blood levels in those instances is quite useless; allergic reactions may even occur after the administration of the drug has already been discontinued, when concentrations are already below the level of detection.

Somewhat in between are some immune phenomena, like the haemolytic anaemia caused by methyldopa. This effect is clearly related to dose and time of exposure, but probably not to the actual concentration at the time this effect is detected. The same hit and run effect can be seen in aspirin thrombopathy: when a patient has a gastric haemorrhage after the use of aspirin, it is more useful to establish his bleeding time than his salicylate level unless one doubts the use of aspirin altogether.

The latter example illustrates an important point, namely that consultation with the laboratory *before* taking samples is often if not always necessary. For the laboratory it often makes a difference whether a qualitative or a quantitative measurement is needed, and whether it is performed on blood or urine. In the above mentioned example this means that a qualitative assay of salicylate in urine may show better whether a patient has taken a salicylate some time before than a serum determination would. In general, drugs that are eliminated mainly in the urine give the clinician the opportunity to assess the total quantity that has been absorbed after ingestion. Of course this can only be done reliably if urine is collected from the moment of admission. Too often the first urine sample is sent to the laboratory for routine tests and then discarded before anybody thinks of its toxicological usefulness.

GUIDANCE OF DRUG THERAPY

A very important reason to determine drug concentrations is for the guidance of drug therapy. Admittedly the need for this is often exaggerated by unexperienced doctors as well as by laboratory specialists, the unexperienced doctor being defined here as the doctor who has not yet learned how to assess the effect of the drug in the patient for whom he prescribed it. For such a doctor, or his patient, a laboratory value is not of much help. As for the laboratory, the supply creates the demand, as is so often the case in clinical medicine. In terms of laboratory organization it is of course more attractive to have a particular drug assay on a routine basis, than to perform it only when really necessary: a car costs less per kilometre the more kilometres driven, but the actual total costs are higher. On the other hand, although one should be warned against the substitution of clinical judgement by drug assays, the undeniable fact that the sensible application of drug assays has enormously contributed to a better treatment of patients should be stressed.

It is important therefore to distinguish between necessary and unnecessary drug assays. The main reason for performing a drug assay for the guidance of therapy is when the result of the treatment is a long-term effect. This applies to the therapeutic as well as to the toxic effects. It has already been mentioned above, that for some drugs it is well-established which concentrations will be toxic to most patients, or at least will aggravate the risk of toxic effects. To give patients the maximal benefit of the drug, the assay of drug concentrations can be of great help. In the past many patients were treated for a long time only to discover that they were not cured after all. It could never be decided whether they were unresponsive to the drug, or whether the drug was not absorbed, or whether it was eliminated too rapidly. Even when drugs are injected, elimination may be variable enough to cause great differences in plasma concentrations.

To establish a rational dosage scheme for an individual patient the actual serum concentrations should be considered in relation to known pharmacokinetic data on the drug. Only then it is relatively easy to adjust the dose, or the dosage interval, or to change the route of administration. Sometimes the dose can be adjusted to a change in renal function by fairly simple calculations, but it is also possible that minor differences between a calculated elimination rate (on the basis of creatinine clearance) and the actual elimination rate lead to great differences between predicted and actual serum levels. It goes without saying that those pharmacokinetic calculations have been made possible only because the fate of drugs in the body, under normal and under pathological conditions has been extensively studied by measuring drugs in body fluids. In short, the most fruitful and effective way to reach the stable drug concentration required as soon as possible, is the "artillery method": calculating for the individual case, aiming, shooting, and adjusting by calculating again. Some gifted people will soon learn how to aim without much calculating and still hit the target. This will be illustrated further in the chapters on anti-arrhythmic drugs, cytostatic drugs, digitalis and antibiotics, the kind of drugs in which assays are particularly helpful because they have a small therapeutic index, or absorption is irregular, or they may accumulate in the body.

CONCLUSION

In conclusion, before a doctor orders a drug assay, he should ask himself what he really wants to know, as precisely as possible: whether he wants the assay for diagnostic reasons, ranging from excluding a not-so-probable diagnosis to confirming a clinically established diagnosis; whether he wants to guide himself during treatment; or whether he wants to enhance his own knowledge of drugs, or even to contribute to the general knowledge of drugs and disease.

REFERENCES

Conn, R.B., Clinical laboratories: profit center, production industry or patient-care resource. *New England Journal of Medicine* 422–427, 454–455 (1978).
Sjöqvist, F., Clinical use of drug plasma level determinations. In: *Yearbook of Drug Therapy.* Ed., Azarnoff, D.A., Hollister, L.E., Shand, D.G., Year Book Medical Publishers, Inc. Chicago–London. 1977, pp. 13–20.

2. RATIONAL SELECTION OF METHODS FOR THERAPEUTIC DRUG MONITORING

D. D. BREIMER

Several considerations may lead to the desirability of monitoring drug concentrations in body fluids of individual patients, if the therapeutic or toxic effect of a certain drug cannot be readily assessed by clinical observation or measurement. These considerations refer either to particular drugs, e.g.:

1. Drugs with a narrow therapeutic ratio (cardiac glycosides);
2. Drugs which show large and unpredictable interindividual variability in drug concentrations from the same dose (tricyclic antidepressants); or to particular clinical situations where in principle any drug may be involved, e.g.:

1. Patients with renal impairment, when the intact drug or its active metabolite(s) undergoes renal excretion to a large extent;
2. Patients with liver disease, when the intact drug or its active metabolite(s) is metabolized to a large extent in the liver;
3. Patients with gastrointestinal disorders, when drugs are given orally and altered absorption may be expected;
4. Patients receiving multiple drug treatment with serious risk of drug interactions;
5. Patients on chronic drug treatment for the verification of compliance;
6. Patients with suspected drug intoxication.

Taking these considerations together means that having a limited number of assays available for a limited number of drugs is not sufficient, but in principle it should be possible to analyse any drug on clinical indication. Although this may not be feasible in rather small clinical settings, it should at least be pursued in the larger and academic hospitals.

DRUG PROPERTIES IN RELATION TO THE ASSAY

If it has been decided that measuring a drug concentration would be useful, the question arises how to do this. For this purpose highly specific and often very sensitive assays for the parent drug and occasionally for its metabolites are required. The rational selection and development of an assay method require special knowledge about the drug to be analysed.

Often isolation of the drug from the biological fluid is involved, followed by a suitable detection procedure.

Physico-chemical properties

A knowledge of the following properties is important:

1. Lipophilicity, to judge whether the compound can be extracted by organic solvents;

2. The pK_a value of acids and bases: it is predominantly the unionized form that travels into the organic solvent and for this reason pH adjustment of the sample prior to extraction may be required;

3. Volatility, to judge whether gas chromatography can be applied, if not, there may be the possibility of rendering the compound volatile by appropriate derivative formation;

4. U.V. absorption, fluorometric and electrochemical characteristics, which will determine the suitability of certain detection techniques for quantitation of the compound;

5. Chemical stability under storage conditions and throughout a particular assay procedure.

Pharmacokinetic properties in man

This information is particularly important to establish the concentration range that should be measured and these ranges may vary widely from drug to drug. In table 1 the therapeutic plasma concentration ranges are given for a number of drugs under steady-state conditions (Sjöqvist et al. 1976). For digoxin, concentrations in the μg/l plasma range are associated with optimal therapy, those for lidocaine are at least a thousandfold higher, whereas salicylate concentrations are a factor of one hundred higher again. Obviously a far more sensitive assay is required for digoxin than for salicylate and at the same time it will be more difficult in the low concentration range to distinguish the compound to be determined from low concentrations of either endogenous or exogenous sample constituents, which makes *selectivity* very important. In other words high sensitivity can only be achieved by a highly selective or specific method.

The concentrations given in table 1 refer to steady-state concentrations. If one is dealing with a single-dose study of a compound with a long half-life,

Table 1. Therapeutic plasma concentration ranges of drugs (mg/l).

Digoxin	0.001–0.002
Nortriptyline	0.050–0.180
Lidocaine	2–5
Phenytoin	10–20
Salicylate	150–300

then obviously far lower concentrations are encountered than during chronic treatment. A more sensitive assay may then be required.

Drug metabolism and pharmacological activity of metabolites in man
Information about the metabolism of a drug is very important, both from an analytical and a therapeutic point of view. The pattern of metabolism, and preferably the physico-chemical and the pharmacological properties of the metabolites, should be known. These may make certain demands upon the selectivity of the method to measure the parent drug and if the metabolites are active, in other words contribute to the overall therapeutic activity, then determining such a metabolite in plasma simultaneously should be considered, e.g. procainamide and N-acetyl-procainamide (de Wolff, this volume, chapter 13), carbamazepine and carbamazepine-epoxide.

The information on the physico-chemical, pharmacokinetic and metabolic properties of a certain drug should be linked with the characteristics of the major analytical techniques which are available for drug assays.

MAJOR TECHNIQUES SUITABLE FOR DRUG MONITORING

The choice of a suitable end-step (actual measurement or detection step) is cardinal to the development of an assay procedure and also largely determines the requirements for sample preparation. The principal techniques and their characteristics are summarized in table 2. For the basic principles of these techniques the reader is referred to textbooks of analytical chemistry.

A major distinction is that certain (spectrophotometric and chromatographic) methods generally require the isolation of the drug from the biological fluid prior to quantitation, whereas in other (immunological) methods the actual measurement takes place in the biological sample itself without cleanup.

Direct U.V. spectrophotometry and spectrofluorometry are not very often applied in therapeutic drug monitoring, due to lack of specificity. However, these detection techniques can be very useful when used in combination with a separation procedure, e.g. thin-layer chromatography or liquid chromatography. The combination of a chromatographic system with a detection system greatly contributes to the selectivity of a particular method, because the chromatographic conditions can be chosen so that there is no interference from metabolites, other drugs or endogenous sample constituents. In gas chromatography selectivity can be improved even more if selective detectors are used, where in particular the nitrogen detector and the electron capture detector have proved very useful, e.g. barbiturates (Breimer and van Rossum 1974), nitrazepam and clonazepam (de Boer et al.

Table 2. Characteristics of analytical techniques.

	Detection limit $(10^{-9}g)$	Separation power (selectivity)	Instrumentation cost ($\times$ 1000 guilders)
U.V. spectrophotometry	100	–	15–60
Spectrofluorometry	1	+ –	20–50
Atomic absorption spectrophotometry	1	+	40–90
Quantitative thin-layer chromatography (densitometry)			
U.V. detection	10	+ +	20–60
Fluorometric detection	1	+ +	20–60
Gas chromatography			
flame ionization detection	1	+ +	20–25
nitrogen selective detection	0.1	+ + +	25–30
Electron capture detection	0.01	+ + +	25–30
Mass fragmentographic detection (GC– MS)	0.001	+ + + +	150–250
Liquid chromatography			
U.V. detection	1	+ +	20–30
Fluorometric detection	0.1	+ + +	30–40
Electrochemical detection	0.01	+ + +	30–40
Immunological methods			
Radioimmunoassay	0.001	+ +	50–80
Enzyme immunoassay	0.001	+ +	25–35
Free radical immunoassay	0.001	+ +	50–100

1978). In fig. 1 an example is given of gas chromatograms obtained after extraction of human plasma containing lidocaine. Pentane was used as extraction solvent (2 $\times$ 5 ml) and N-methylhexobarbital was added as internal standard. The gas chromatographic column was a capillary SCOT (support-coated open tubular) column and detection occurred with a nitrogen detector. The figure illustrates that if the combination of a good separation system with a highly selective detection technique is applied, the extraction procedure can be very simple and still achieve great sensitivity. Similar results may be obtained with liquid chromatography, although the more sensitive and selective detection techniques, e.g. polarography, are still in a state of development. In fig. 2 an example is given of a chromatogram obtained after extraction of human plasma containing theophylline.

The most specific and sensitive technique presently available is still gas chromatography combined with mass spectrometry, where the intensity of certain specific mass fragments is a measure for the concentration of the compound to be assayed (Millard 1976). However, this instrument is very expensive and requires considerable skill. Although it is almost indispens-

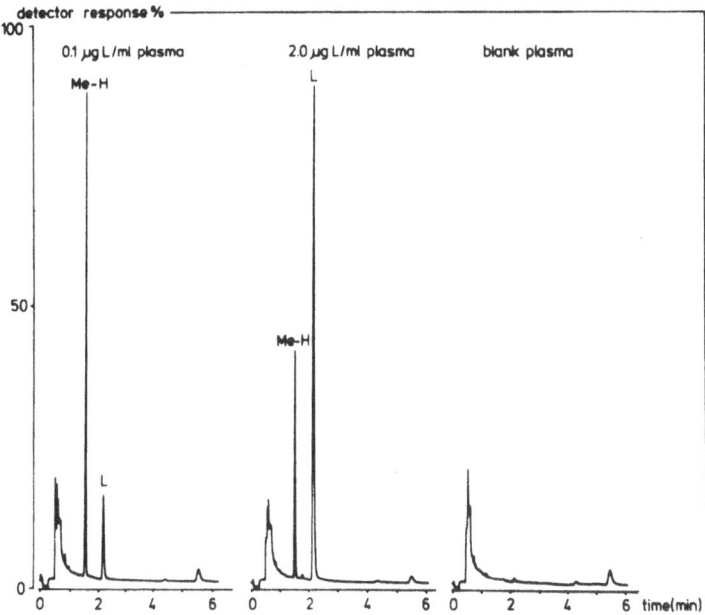

Figure 1. Gas chromatographic determination of lidocaine in human plasma. *Right*: a gas chromatogram obtained after extraction of blank plasma with N-pentane. *Left and centre:* after extraction of plasma to which known amounts of lidocaine (L) had been added. N-Methylhexobarbital (Me-H) was used as internal standard. Conditions: SCOT column; i.d., 0.40 mm; length, 10 m; coating, Carbowax 20M; temp., 160°C; helium, 10 ml/min; solid injection system; nitrogen detector (De Boer et al., in press).

able for laboratories involved in pharmacokinetic and drug metabolism research, it is certainly not an instrument with wide application in the field of therapeutic drug monitoring.

When it comes to the question of convenience of an assay attention should be paid to the immunoassays, which have been developed and improved for a number of drugs in recent years. The great advantage is that the actual measurement of the compound to be analysed takes place in small samples, without prior isolation. In radioimmunoassay detection takes place by radioactivity measurement in a liquid scintillation or gamma counter (Landon and Moffat 1976). Disadvantages are the licensing requirements for working with radioactive material and the rather expensive detection system. A newer and most promising development, however, in the field of immunoassays is the so-called enzyme immunoassay, where the detection label is not a radio-active isotope but an enzyme covalently bound to the drug to be assayed (Scharpé et al. 1976). If the drug-enzyme conjugate is not bound to the antibody, the enzyme retains its capacity to convert its natural substrate. The amount of substrate converted can be followed by a relatively simple spectrophotometer, e.g., in the cases where glucose-6-

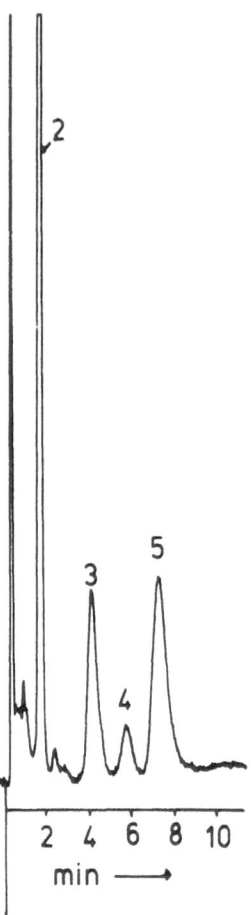

Figure 2. HPLC determination of theophylline and coffeine metabolites in human plasma. Chromatogram obtained after extraction of blank plasma with ether/dichloromethane (7:4); 2 = coffeine; 3 = theobromine; 4 = theophylline (here as a metabolite of coffeine); 5 = paraxanthine. Stationary phase: silicagel SI 60 (Mereck); mobile phase: 1% of a solution of ammoniumformiate (0.020%) and formic acid (0.017%) on methanol (Danhof et al., 1978).

phosphate dehydrogenase is the enzyme, and nicotine adenine dinucleotide is used as the coenzyme.

The reliability of any immunoassay obviously depends very much on the specificity of the antibody towards the drug to be determined. Any compound, part of whose molecule is identical or closely similar to the antigenic determinant part of the drug, will compete for antibody binding sites and influence the results with drugs. Such interference may arise from the presence of metabolites or other drugs with structural similarities. For example with the digoxin antibodies, which were available some years ago, interference with the frequently co-administered structurally related diuretic spironolactone was encountered (Zeegers et al. 1973). Cross-reactivity with metabolites and other drugs should always be determined when using a particular immunoassay (van Oostveen, 1976; Drost et al. 1977).

An important check for the specificity of the antibody is a correlation study with a specific chemical method, if available. In the case of digoxin this is almost impossible, but for the anti-epileptic drugs this can readily be done. An example is given in fig. 3, for phenytoin, where gas chromatography and radioimmunoassay are compared (Orme et al., 1976).

It can be expected that the combination of sensitivity, specificity, and convenience of the assay procedure that characterizes immunoassay will be employed to an increasing extent in the quantitative determination of drug levels in biological fluids. However, one has to be aware of cross-reactions with other compounds and realize that the precision and accuracy of

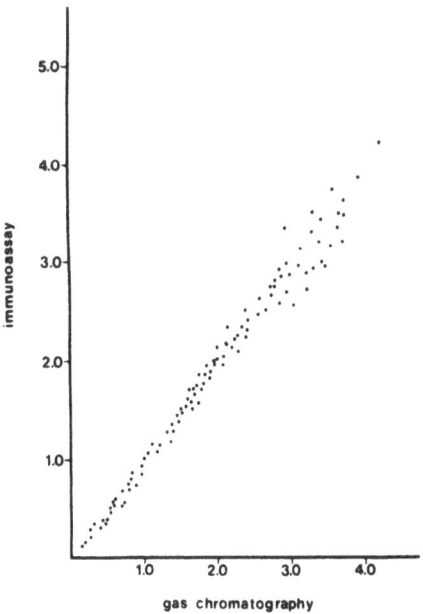

Figure 3. Comparison between plasma phenytoin (DPH) concentrations (μg/ml) as measured by gas chromatography and radioimmunoassay in 105 samples taken from six patients with impaired renal function (Orme et al. 1976).

most immunoassays may not approach those of a good chemical or chromatographic method. These assays should not be run at the limits of sensitivity
and rigid quality control should be exercised.

CRITERIA FOR SELECTION OF A PARTICULAR METHOD

Detection limit and sensitivity
The detection limit depends largely on the actual detection technique
(table 2) but is also determined by the biological sample size. For instance, it
may be very well possible to determine a drug concentration of 100 μg/l
plasma by gas chromatography in a 2-ml plasma sample obtained from an
adult patient. However, this may become rather difficult if only 0.1 ml
samples from children or infants are available. A more sensitive method,
e.g. immunoassay, may then be required.

Accuracy and specificity
An accurate method for a particular drug measures exactly the concentration of this drug in the biological sample when it was taken. There
should be no interference from metabolites, other drugs or endogenous
sample constituents and there should be no other systematic errors. Often
this requires the combination of an extraction procedure and a chromatographic separation step, followed by a selective detection technique. In
practice this cannot always be achieved; sometimes a rapid assay with
limited specificity may be more useful for an acute clinical situation than a
very accurate time-consuming method.

Precision (reproducibility)
Any method used in drug monitoring should be as precise as possible.
Although this may seem a superfluous statement, it is surprising to notice
sometimes the great differences in results obtained by different people
running exactly the same assay for exactly the same sample (Dijkhuis
1975; Pippenger et al. 1976; Richens, this volume). Efforts should be made
to achieve high inter-technician and interlaboratory reproducibility by
means of participation in quality control schemes.

Convenience and cost of the assay
These aspects are especially important when routine multiple sample assays
are required. Time of sample preparation, instrumentation cost, automation
possibilities, which are now available for many techniques, have to be considered. In this respect the immunoassays are particularly attractive, because
they do not require laborious sample preparation. Convenience and low

cost may, however, sometimes have to be at the expense of the desired accuracy.

WHAT BIOLOGICAL FLUID SHOULD BE ANALYSED?

In principle any biological fluid could be used, but in practice plasma or serum, whole blood, saliva, urine, and sometimes cerebrospinal fluid are sampled.

Plasma or serum
This is the most commonly used fluid for drug assays. It is assumed that particularly during chronic drug treatment (steady-state conditions) drug concentration at the site of action is closely related to that in plasma. Moreover, the therapeutic plasma concentration range has been established for a number of drugs (table 1).

Whole blood
For most drugs concentration in plasma is proportional to that in erythrocytes, so that measuring whole blood concentration offers no additional information. Exceptions are represented by drugs which are considerably bound to erythrocytes and the kinetics of which differ from that in plasma, e.g. chlorthalidone (Fleuren and van Rossum 1975).

Saliva
The observation that drug concentrations in saliva are often proportional to the concentrations in plasma has led to the suggestion that in therapeutic drug monitoring, or in pharmacokinetic studies in general, saliva might be substituted for plasma. Saliva can be obtained by non-invasive techniques, generally following the stimulation of salivary flow by chewing on some semi-solid material or by spraying citric acid on the tongue.

There is evidence that many organic compounds enter saliva by a passive diffusion process, where lipid solubility and the degree of ionization, dependent on plasma and salivary pH, are important factors. In addition, it has been shown for some drugs that their concentration in saliva equals the free or protein-unbound concentration in plasma, which is an advantage because drug plasma concentrations generally represent both bound and unbound drug. If saliva is to be used in therapeutic monitoring then the saliva-to-plasma concentration ratio should be constant over a wide plasma concentration range. For a number of anticonvulsant drugs and for digoxin a quite consistent correlation between their concentrations in saliva and plasma has been established under steady-state conditions (fig. 4). Many drugs have not been sufficiently studied during continuous treatment, whereas in

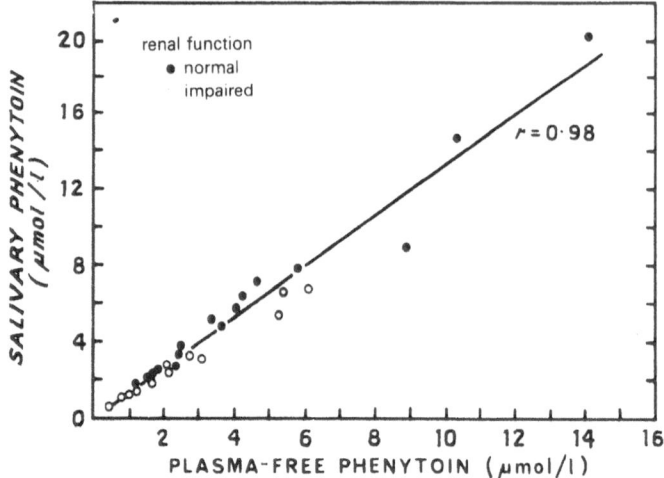

Figure 4. Salivary and plasma-free phenytoin concentrations in epileptics with normal and impaired renal function (Reynolds et al. 1976).

single dose studies great discrepancies in saliva/plasma ratio have been observed. For a review on the use of saliva in therapeutic drug monitoring see Danhof and Breimer (1978).

In principle, the analytical procedures which have been developed for the assay of drugs in plasma are equally suitable for drug monitoring in saliva. However, salivary concentrations of some highly protein-bound drugs are far lower than plasma concentrations, which may require modification of existing procedures or development of more sensitive methods.

Urine
The concentration of unchanged drug in urine does not directly reflect the concentration of the drug in plasma, since it is the urinary excretion *rate* that is proportional to the plasma concentration. This means that for therapeutic drug monitoring purposes a single urine concentration is of no value. It should further be realized that many drugs are excreted unchanged into urine only in negligible amounts. Obviously urine sampling can be very interesting for certain pharmacokinetic, bioavailability or drug metabolism investigations. It is very useful for checking drug compliance qualitatively and for identification purposes in intoxication cases.

SAMPLE COLLECTION AND STORAGE

Specific problems and pitfalls may be associated with biological sample collection and the storage of the sample until it is analysed. The use of certain syringes, canules or tubes may cause either loss of drug due to absorption into plastic or release of plasticizers into the biological medium, which will interfere with the assay. For propranolol a redistribution phenomenon between plasma and erythrocytes has been reported, which was caused by the release of certain substances from tube stoppers (Cotham and Shand 1975). Saliva collection often takes place by stimulating salivary flow by chewing parafilm, which may absorb lipophilic drugs (Chang and Chiou 1976). The storage conditions should be checked for decomposition of the compounds to be analysed. Clonazepam in plasma, for example, decomposes readily at room temperature, but is stable at 4°C for long periods (Knop et al. 1975). An aspect that is generally not taken into account, but which may occasionally be important is that whole blood is collected at 37°C, but plasma and serum are generally separated at lower temperatures. If drug erythrocyte binding and plasma protein binding are temperature-dependent, and this is generally the case, then the drug concentration in plasma after centrifugation may be different from that at 37°C (Ehrnebo and Odar-Cederlöf 1977). It is in any case recommended to collect blood and separate plasma under standardized conditions.

CONCLUSIONS

Many analytical techniques, some with highly developed technology, can be be used for the quantitative determination of almost any drug and its metabolites in biological fluids. It depends on the objective of the assay (e.g. research, therapy, intoxication) which criterion will determine the ultimate choice. For therapeutic monitoring of specific single drugs, immunoassays may provide the sensitivity, selectivity, precision, and particularly the rapidity and convenience, needed for the performance of large numbers of drug analyses on small volumes of plasma or saliva. However, improvements are still required with respect to the specificity and precision which can be achieved with the currently available kits.

Other (chromatographic) techniques are essential for the therapeutic monitoring of drugs in general, and for all kinds of pharmacokinetic, metabolism and bioavailability studies in man. It is at the same time very important that those who are responsible for these types of assay should have a profound knowledge of not only analytical chemistry and methods – that is certainly not sufficient in the context of the problems involved – but also of *drugs*, their physico-chemical properties, their pharmacology, their therapeutic action, their fate in the body and their metabolism. Only in such a context has a drug assay perspective and can it be of real value for the optimal treatment of an individual patient.

REFERENCES

De Boer, A.G., Röst-Kaiser, J., Bracht, H. and Breimer, D.D., Assay of underivatized nit-
    razepam and clonazepam in plasma by capillary gas chromatography applied for
    pharmacokinetic and bioavailability studies in man. *Journal of Chromatography: Biome-
    dical Applications* 145, 105–114 (1978).
de Boer, A.G., Breimer, D.D. and Mattie, H., Rectal bioavailability of lidocaine from a
    suppository and a slow release preparation in man. *Pharmaceutisch Weekblad*, in press.
Breimer, D.D. and van Rossum, J.M., Rapid and sensitive gas chromatographic determina-
    tion of hexobarbital in plasma of man using a nitrogen detector. *Journal of Chromato-
    graphy* 88, 235–243 (1974).
Chang, K. and Chiou, W.L., Interactions between drugs and saliva-stimulating parafilm and
    their implications in measurements of saliva drug levels. *Research Communications in
    Chemical Pathology and Pharmacology* 13, 357–360 (1976).
Cotham, R.H. and Shand, D. Spuriously low plasma propranolol concentrations resulting
    from blood collection methods. *Clinical Pharmacology and Therapeutics* 18, 535–538
    (1975).
Danhof, M. and Breimer, D.D.: Therapeutic drug monitoring in saliva. *Clinical Pharma-
    cokinetics* 3, 39–57 (1978).
Danhof, M., Loomans, B.M.J. and Breimer, D.D., Bepaling van theophylline in plasma en
    speeksel, in aanwezigheid van coffeïnemetabolieten, met behulp van HPLC. *Pharma-
    ceutisch Weekblad* 113, 672–676 (1978).
Dijkhuis, I.C., Interlaboratoriumonderzoek naar de bepaling van anti-epileptica in plasma
    of serum met behulp van gelyofiliseerd standaardplasma. *Pharmaceutisch Weekblad*
    110, 1177–1199 (1975).
Drost, R.H., Plomp, T.A., Teunissen, A.J., Maas, A.H.J. and Maes, R.A.A., A comparative
    study of the homogeneous enzyme immunoassay (Emit) and two radioimmunoassays
    (RIA's) for digoxin. *Clinica Chimica Acta* 79, 557–567 (1977).
Ehrnebo, M. and Odar-Cederlöf, I., Distribution of pentobarbital and diphenylhydantoin
    between plasma and cells in blood: effect of salicylic acid, temperature and total drug
    concentration. *European Journal of Clinical Pharmacology* 11, 37–42 (1977).
Fleuren, H.L.J.M. and van Rossum, J.M., Pharmacokinetics of chlorthalidone in man.
    Pharmaceutisch Weekblad 110, 1262–1264 (1975).
Knop, H.J., van der Kleijn, E. and Edmunds, L.C., The determination of clonazepam in
    plasma by gas liquid chromatography. *Pharmaceutisch Weekblad* 110, 297–309 (1975).
Landon, J. and Moffat, A.C., The radioimmunoassay of drugs. *The Analyst* 101, 225–243
    (1976).
Millard, B.J., Newer developments in the mass spectrometry of drugs and metabolites.
    In: *Progress in Drug Metabolism*, vol. 1. Ed. *Bridges, J.W. and Chasseud, L.F.* London,
    1976, pp. 1–39.
van Oostveen, J.J.J., De kwantitatieve bepaling van digoxine in biologisch materiaal: II:
    Radioimmunoassay. *Pharmaceutisch Weekblad* 111, 45–53 (1976).
Orme, M.L'E., Borgå, O., Cook, C.E. and Sjöqvist, F., Measurement of diphenylhydantoin
    in 0.1-ml plasma samples: gas chromatography and radioimmunoassay compared.
    Clinical Chemistry 22, 246–249 (1976).
Pippenger, C., Penry, J.K., White, B.G., Daly, D.D. and Buddington, R., Interlaboratory
    variability in determination of plasma anti-epileptic drug concentration. *Archives of
    Neurology* 33, 351–355 (1976).
Reynolds, F., Ziroyanis, P.N., Jones, N.F. and Smith, S.E., Salivary phenytoin concentrations
    in epilepsy and in chronic renal failure. *Lancet* ii, 384–386 (1976).
Scharpé, S.L., Cooreman, W.M., Blomme, W.J. and Laekeman, G.M., Quantitative enzyme
    immunoassay. *Clinical Chemistry* 22, 733–738 (1976).
Sjöqvist, F., Borgå, O. and Orme, M.L'E., Fundamentals of clinical pharmacology. In:
    Drug Treatment. Ed., Avery, G.S., ADIS-Press, Sydney, 1976, p. 32.
Zeegers, J.J.W., Maas, A.H.J., Willebrands, A.F., Kruijswijk, H.H. and Jambroes, G., The
    radioimmunoassay of plasma-digoxin. *Clinica Chimica Acta* 44, 109–116 (1973).

General Reading

Brodie, B.B., Gillette, J.R. and Ackerman, H.S., eds., *Handbook of Experimental Pharmacology*, vol. 28, part 2: *Concepts in Biochemical Pharmacology*, Berlin, 1971.

Ciba Foundation Symposium, *The Poisoned Patient: the Role of the Laboratory*, Amsterdam, 1974.

Garrett, E.R. and Hirtz. J.L., eds., *Drug Fate and Metabolism*, vols. 1, 2, New York, 1977–1978.

Reid, E., ed., *Assay of Drugs and Other Trace Compounds in Biological Fluids*, Amsterdam, 1976.

3. MANAGEMENT OF A CLINICAL DRUG LABORATORY

F.A. DE WOLFF

This book is primarily intended for clinicians wishing to enlarge their knowledge in the field of practical therapeutics, but there are two obvious reasons for inserting a chapter on laboratory management. First, some knowledge of specific laboratory problems may lead to a better understanding between the clinician and the laboratory staff, and, therefore, to more carefully thought-out requests to the laboratory. Secondly, a number of readers may not yet have extensive laboratory facilities for drug determinations at their disposal, but are probably planning to request that their hospital management set up such a service. We will try to provide those courageous people with some information which may be valuable in their endeavours. Thereby we shall, rather immodestly, use our own laboratory, the toxicology laboratory of Leiden's university hospital, as an example, although one must realize that our structure is not necessarily the only correct one.

CONTACT BETWEEN CLINICIAN AND LABORATORY

As with everything in clinical practice, drug determinations are performed for the benefit of the patient, and in particular to establish an individual therapeutic scheme. Usually, there is no direct contact between the patient and the laboratory – the interaction between them is shown schematically in fig. 1. It is obvious that the clinician plays a central role in this contact. In this chapter we will confine ourselves to the second step in this scheme: the contacts between the clinician and the laboratory, and, in addition, to the needs which should be met by an efficiently working drug laboratory. Physical examination and case history are the privilege of the clinician, and laboratory analysis is the competence of the laboratory specialist. The indication for the performance of drug assays and the interpretation of the laboratory results into clinically relevant data are, however, both matters for dialogue between the physician and the laboratory staff. Since the present generation of doctors is not yet trained to interpret the results of drug assays, and since clinical indications for the determination of drugs in body fluids of patients are increasing, this type of dialogue will be more and more an integral part of patient care. For instance, in a patient a certain type of epilepsy is diagnosed and carbamazepine is prescribed. On the second day of treatment,

F.A. DE WOLFF

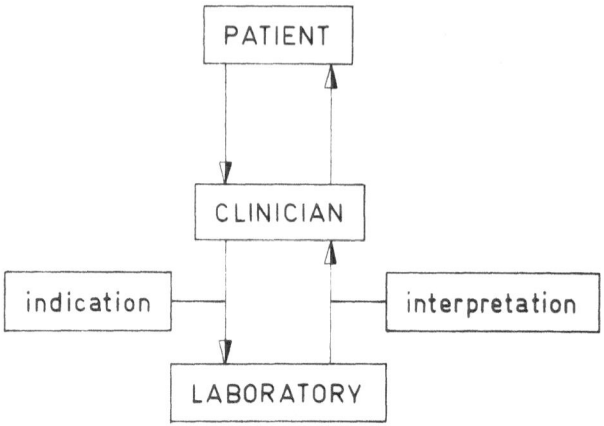

Figure 1. Interaction between the patient and the clinical drug laboratory.

the neurologist asks the laboratory specialist whether it is useful to determine a serum level of the drug. The answer should be that it depends upon the clinical situation. If the patient is not free from fits and one just wants to know whether or not he takes the drug or it is absorbed, then the assay should be performed. However, since carbamazepine has an initial serum half-life of approximately two days and because generally no loading dose is given, it will take at least a week before the patient has reached a steady-state serum level. The present example is complicated by the fact that carbamazepine may accelerate its own metabolism by liver enzyme induction, and therefore the neurologist must also be informed that the assay should be repeated after a week, and again after several weeks, even if the patient reacts well to the medication. If he does not, earlier analysis is, of course, indicated to decide whether or not carbamazepine is the right choice of drug for this patient.

In many cases it will not be necessary to consult the laboratory staff personally. The request to the laboratory can then be done simply by completing the appropriate form. The laboratory form should be clearly recognizable as intended for drug assays, and, to avoid irritation, it should not be too complicated to fill in. It must be considered as the visiting card of the laboratory and should have space for the following relevant details:

1. Patient identification;
2. Doctor, ward, date, telephone number;
3. Sample (blood, urine, stomach contents, saliva);
4. Drug(s) to be assayed;
5. Dosage scheme;
6. Times of last medication and of sampling; and
7. Other drugs prescribed.

It should be stressed that a serum level without this additional knowledge gives no relevant information. Although the laboratory form is very important, it is more important to realize that it must never be the only means of communication between the clinician and the laboratory. The form should never fully replace personal contact, to prevent the *laboratory* doctor from becoming a *paper* doctor. Personal contact is also necessary to avoid the drug laboratory suffering from the disease which I call "Sorcerer's Apprentice Syndrome" in clinical chemistry. As soon as the contact between clinician and drug laboratory specialist occurs only via computer terminals, the number of requests will increase enormously and lead to a huge amount of unnecessary determinations, which, like the water in Goethe's ballad, can hardly ever be reduced. Automation and more computerization in the drug laboratory will become unavoidable; for economic reasons the sending of more samples will be advocated, and so on. Both clinicians and laboratory specialists should be well aware of the dangers of a too technocratic development. Therefore, good contact between the clinician and the laboratory specialist should be nursed.

As soon as the assay is performed, the result has to be interpreted. For instance, when the drug concentration in the aforementioned carbamazepine example remains too low with respect to the prescribed dose, we must try to find the cause. This may be either liver enzyme induction or non-compliance, or a number of other things. In my opinion, the laboratory specialist should give complementary information to the clinician. For instance, when our carbamazepine patient happens to be a woman taking oral contraceptives and there is any indication of liver enzyme induction, then the clinician should be advised that low-dose oral contraception is no longer reliable, and that it should be adjusted.

From the point of view of a laboratory specialist, the doctors who consult the laboratory can be divided roughly into four types, analogous to the four sons referred to in the Passover Haggadah in which the exodus of the people of Israel from Egypt is described (fig. 2). First, there is the junior doctor who has just passed his examinations. He is too young even to ask questions and should, therefore, be educated in practical therapeutics from the beginning. Secondly there is the simple doctor. He has been working in practical medicine for years, but he still believes that phenobarbital is a short-acting hypnotic. Discussions with him are time-consuming and usually without effect. As a matter of fact, this type is rare. Thirdly there is the bad doctor. He does not ask questions; he just gives commands to the laboratory, such as: "I have a patient on diazepam and I need a serum concentration within the hour." Fortunately, this type is also rare. And last but not least, there is the wise doctor who poses only well-considered requests, and with whom every discussion is pleasant and fruitful.]

Up till now, we have discussed how the clinician should behave, but we have said nothing so far about the laboratory specialist. I think it is difficult

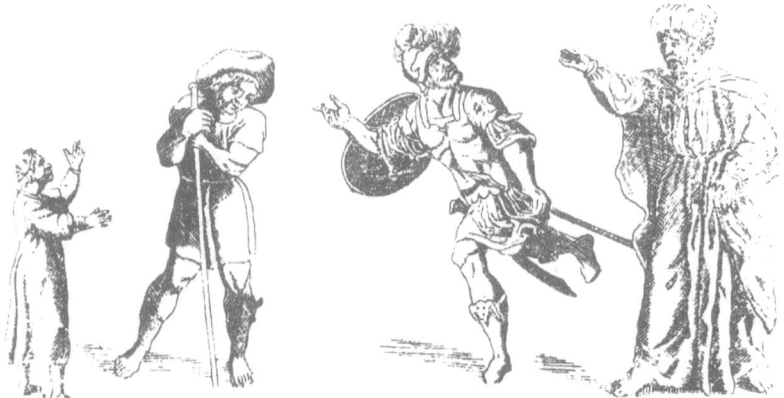

Figure 2.   The four sons, from a Dutch Haggadah of 1881 (de Vries 1968).

to give a profile of the ideal laboratory doctor. He should, first of all, have a profound knowledge of pharmacology, both general and clinical, and be able to speak and understand the language of the clinician. He should also be an expert in clinical and analytical chemistry to evaluate existing laboratory methods and to develop new ones. There is no academic training for a "drug laboratory doctor," and in my opinion such a study would be impossible because of the divergent character of the job. Since nobody can combine all these abilities in one person, the most ideal situation would be a staff of at least two scientists: one clinical pharmacologist and one chemical or pharmaceutical graduate who specialized in drug analysis. In view of these facts it is rather irrelevant that some specific professional groups claim to be experts in the management of drug laboratories.

LABORATORY METHODOLOGY

We have dealt so far with the aspects of indication and interpretation, but after the indication has been defined and before interpretation can be given, the assay has to be performed. The analysis is, of course, very important. The therapeutic relevance of a poor analysis is nil. The chemical determination can be compared with the X-ray photograph of the radiologist: it is not the whole story, but it is the technical foundation upon which conclusions are based. Therefore, the laboratory results should be as reliable as possible.

For the analytical work there are three basic needs: *space*, *equipment* and *staff*. It is commonplace to say that in these difficult times it is not easy to lay hands on these three essentials, and everyone who wants to set up a drug laboratory nowadays has to fight hard. The manner in which such a battle can be fought could be the subject of another chapter, but is beyond the scope of this book.

The space necessary is dependent on the programme of the laboratory, the equipment that can be obtained and the number of staff available. As for the analytical equipment in the drug laboratory, the absolute minimum should be at least two gas chromatographs and a spectrophotometer. In a larger centre, more gas chromatographs with different detectors must be present, preferably one for every column that is currently used. In addition an atomic absorption spectrophotometer with flame and graphite furnace should be present. High-pressure liquid chromatography is a promising technique, although it can as yet not replace gas chromatography. Thin-layer chromatography (TLC) is not only indispensable for qualitative work; thanks to the development of specific thin-layer densitometers it can also be used as a quantitative technique, especially for those drugs that are thermo-labile in the gas chromatograph. Another advantage is that with this technique the analyst has a visual check: the determined drug is not only represented by a peak on a recorder, but also by a coloured or fluorescent spot on the thin-layer plate. Recent developments, for instance the manufacturing of plates with concentration zones and of high-performance thin-layer plates, as well as the construction of better densitometers, may be very important for drug analysis in the near future. Immunoassays are also becoming more and more important. Since enzyme immunoassays are gradually superseding radio-immunoassays, the liquid scintillation counter will probably be replaced by a multipurpose spectrophotometer. Fluorometry is a dying technique: it is very sensitive to drugs, but also to many interfering substances from the glassware or the bench. In my opinion, a drug laboratory can work perfectly without a cuvette fluorometer. However, fluorometry as a detection system in liquid and thin-layer chromatography is very promising.

Since drug determinations are usually rather complicated, one should make high demands on the equipment and buy the very best available. The same goes for the technical staff, although they cannot be bought. Technicians should have qualifications of the highest level, since the work in the drug laboratory is not simple, and can by no means be compared with the determinations of haemoglobin, sodium and potassium in the average clinical laboratory. One technician only in the drug laboratory is insufficient: if he becomes ill or goes on holiday, there is nobody left. For a laboratory providing both a round-the-clock toxicology service and a service for therapeutic drug monitoring, at least three highly qualified technicians are needed.

As for the nature of techniques to be chosen, the golden rule is: let them be as simple as possible. Even the most simple drug determination is complicated enough. When our laboratory took over the therapeutic monitoring of anticonvulsant drugs a few years ago, it also took over the other laboratory's technique. The chromatographic system proved to be excellent, but the extraction step was extremely complicated, with much personal witchcraft (Driessen and Emonds 1974), and the results were rather fluctuating. Then I visited the Poisons Unit at Guy's Hospital in London, and one of the many interesting things I learned there was the direct injection method without evaporation of the solvent used for extraction of the drugs from the sample (Flanagan and Berry 1977). We modified the anticonvulsant assay according to this very simple principle and since then the results have been more reliable.

QUALITY CONTROL

The only way to check your results in an objective manner is by participation in a quality control scheme. It should be stressed that working without quality control is irresponsible. There are two possible quality control methods: *internal* and *external*, both of which should be used. Internal quality control means that in every series of samples one serum with a known content of the drug is included, so that it can be ascertained whether the laboratory is having a bad day, in which case the technician should, of course, start again. This system is not very objective. Internal quality control is only useful in establishing day-to-day variations, and variations between different technicians. Therefore, external quality control is always indicated in addition to internal quality control. A good example of an external quality control scheme is the one organized for anticonvulsant drugs from St. Bartholomew's Hospital in London by A. Richens, in which eight Dutch laboratories participate at present. A set of specimens, usually aliquots of a pool made from patients' serum, is mailed each month to each laboratory. The samples are analysed and the results are sent back to London, where statistical analysis is carried out. For each type of assay and for each laboratory a computer print-out is made (Richens, this volume) and sent to the participants. From the histogram, the standard deviation and the coefficient of variation, the results can be compared with those of others. In addition to this international quality control scheme, a quality control system is organized in Holland by I.C. Dijkhuis of the The Hague Hospital Pharmacies. This organization offers programmes for anticonvulsants, cardiac drugs, and toxicology.

Participation in a quality control scheme is also very important for the self-confidence of the laboratory specialist. Every clinical chemist has experience with the doctor who tells him regularly: "I have the impression that your calciums are a little too low these last few weeks". When asked for proof, the doctor just answers: "I have no proof, I have just the impression." When the laboratory can show him favourable results of a quality control programme, he will be readily convinced that not the calciums but his impressions were wrong.

EXTENT OF SERVICE

When setting up a drug laboratory, the question arises as to what the extent of the service should be. A list of drugs of which the determination in plasma or serum has been shown to be of direct therapeutic value is given in table 1. A survey of toxicologically important drug determinations is given by van Heijst in chapter 17. A drug laboratory in a large medical centre should, in principle, be able to measure most drugs and toxic substances not only for therapeutic monitoring, but also to check, for instance, non-compliance or forbidden drug intake. But what about a smaller hospital? If the requests for a drug determination remain below a certain level, then the samples could better be sent to a larger centre with more experience. This minimum level differs from drug to drug. If the total amount of requests for phenytoin remains below, say, one per week, it is not worthwhile setting up a phenytoin monitoring service, because the laboratory specialist will probably never get enough experience with the assay and the interpretation of the results. With other types of drugs, this minimum level may be much lower. For instance, in our laboratory phenprocoumon and acenocoumarol, the coumarin anticoagulants used in The Netherlands, are assayed, and since indications for these determinations are rather rare, specimens are sent to us from all over the country. In spite of this, the total requests do not exceed four assays a month. Although this does not seem economical, which indeed it is not, we continue to perform these assays because we are one of the few laboratories which have a little experience with them.

On the other hand, we have no experience whatsoever, for instance, in arsenic poisoning, so when a patient suspected of arsenic poisoning is admitted, about three times a year, we gladly send his urine to a colleague who is more experienced in this field.

Table 1. Drugs for which determination in serum has direct therapeutic value.

Antiepileptics	Cardiac drugs	Psychotropic drugs	Miscellaneous
Carbamazepine	Digoxin	Desipramine	Antibiotics
Clonazepam	Lidocaine	Imipramine	Isoniazide
Dipropylacetate	Procainamide	Lithium	Methotrexate
(Valproate)	Quinidine	Nortriptyline	Sulfonamides
Ethosuximide			Theophylline
Phenobarbital			
Phenytoin			

COST-BENEFIT

With the economic side of the matter I must be brief, since I am no econo-
mist. From data obtained in our laboratory, where four to five thousand
assays are performed each year, we can calculate that the average overall
cost of one drug determination is about one hundred guilders. This seems
very expensive, but we must realize that one day in hospital for one patient
costs three times as much. It is obvious that when a patient is hospitalized
longer than necessary because drug determinations are not performed,
money is being wasted.

CONCLUSIONS

A clinical drug laboratory should be headed by a laboratory specialist
who has a thorough knowledge of both pharmacology and the analytical
chemistry of drugs. He should be assisted by at least two qualified technicians. Gas chromatography and spectrophotometry are the most important
techniques in the drug laboratory. For the evaluation of the results, the
laboratory should participate in an external quality control programme.
Intensive contact between the laboratory staff and the clinician is indispensable for efficient functioning of the laboratory.

REFERENCES

Driessen, O. and Emonds, A., Simultaneous determination of anti-epileptic drugs in small
    samples of blood plasma by gas chromatography: column technology and extraction
    procedure. *Proc. Kon. Ned. Acad. Wetensch.*, Series C, 77, 171–181 (1974).
Flanagan, R.J. and Berry, D.J., Routine analysis of barbiturates and some other hypnotic
    drugs in the blood plasma as an aid to the diagnosis of acute poisoning. *Journal of
    Chromatography* 133, 131–146 (1977).
De Vries, S.P., *Joodse riten en symbolen*, Amsterdam, 1968.

4. CLINICAL RELEVANCE OF SERUM DRUG LEVEL MONITORING, WITH PARTICULAR REFERENCE TO PHENYTOIN

A. RICHENS

When a drug is administered to a patient, a certain serum concentration will result which produces a tissue effect whose magnitude is determined by the serum concentration. Since we have been able to measure serum drug concentrations, we have realized that with most drugs there is a wide intersubject variation in the serum concentration produced by a standard dose of drug, such that some patients will have a level well below the accepted range while others will have a toxic level. This variation is caused by differences in the absorption, distribution and elimination of the drug, factors which are collectively called *pharmacokinetic factors*, and variation in these is called *pharmacokinetic variation* (Fig. 1). The factors which determine the relationship between the serum level and the resulting pharmacological effect are called *pharmacodynamic factors*, and variation in these is called *pharmacodynamic variation*. Although the latter has been studied far less than pharmacokinetic variation, it is generally thought to be less important, If this assumption is correct, it follows that monitoring serum drug concentrations in order to tailor the dose to suit the individual's need will largely overcome the problem of differences in response to drugs.

There are an increasing number of drugs for which serum level monitoring would appear to be of value. Prominent amongst these are the antiepileptic drugs, lithium, antidysrhythmic drugs, digoxin, theophylline, aminoglycoside antibiotics and tricyclic antidepressants. Perhaps the most

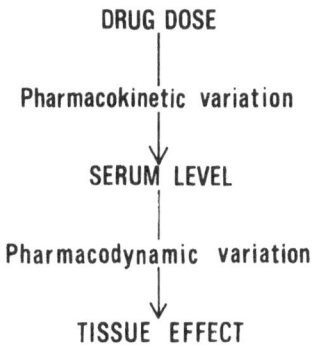

Figure 1. Variation in response to drugs.

studied drug has been phenytoin, and therefore this compound will be used to illustrate the purpose of this paper, namely to explore the clinical relevance of drug monitoring.

BENEFITS OF DRUG MONITORING

Phenytoin is a particularly good example of a drug for which a pharmacokinetic approach is essential if it is to be used correctly. Serum levels vary widely in patients receiving standard doses; the drug has a narrow therapeutic ratio; the relationship between dose and serum level is non-linear because its metabolism is saturable and therefore dose adjustments need to take this into account; and lastly, problems of non-compliance, generic inequivalence, and drug interactions are common. Traditionalists argue that the proper way to use the drug is to increase the dose gradually until control of fits is reached or until adverse effects become dose-limiting, thus tailoring the dose according to the patient's response. However, in practice this approach has not worked well. Many surveys have shown that serum levels in epileptic outpatients are scattered widely from subtherapeutic to toxic, and individual values do not appear to have been adjusted to obtain optimum control. Indeed, Koch-Weser (1975) in his survey at the Massachusetts General Hospital showed that over ninety percent of patients were receiving the standard dose of one capsule of Dilantin (100 mg) three times daily, even though only twenty-seven percent had serum levels within the accepted therapeutic range.

Failure of therapy on standard doses of one drug is usually followed by addition of a second drug, and perhaps later a third. Shorvon and Reynolds (1977) reviewed retrospectively the pattern of prescribing in their own epilepsy clinic at King's College Hospital, London, and remarked on the frequency with which a second drug had been added prematurely before an attempt to optimize the dose of the first had been made. The same group found in a prospective study that if the dose of phenytoin was tailored by monitoring serum levels, more than ninety per cent of newly presenting outpatients were controlled by this one drug alone (Reynolds et al. 1976). Previously, almost two thirds of them would have been put on a second drug. A follow-up report has shown that most patients have continued to respond favourably, and that carbamazepine used as sole therapy is equally effective (Shorvon et al. 1978).

Undoubtedly then, monitoring serum phenytoin levels is invaluable in tailoring the dose to suit the patient. If this information is to be used correctly, however, a sound knowledge of phenytoin kinetics is necessary, particularly an understanding of the saturable nature of its metabolism. The capacity of hepatic microsomal enzymes to hydroxylate phenytoin is limited, so that over the therapeutic range of serum levels the rate of metabolism does not rise in proportion with the serum level, as is usual with most drugs (whose metabolism obeys *first order kinetics*). Eventually the capacity to metabolize phenytoin is completely saturated and a fixed amount of the drug is removed in a given time, regardless of how high the serum level becomes (a situation described as *zero order kinetics*).

The consequence of this type of kinetics in man is that a non-linear relationship exists between dose and serum level (fig. 2). Unit increments in dose produce progressively larger increments in serum level such that an increase of 50 mg or less may be sufficient to raise the serum level from subtherapeutic to toxic (Richens 1975b; Richens and Dunlop 1975a). I have seen a number of patients in whom a dose increase appears to have been made on the assumption that a linear dose/level relationship exists, and the result has been gross intoxication (Richens et al. 1976).

For drugs that show first order kinetics, an accurate prediction of the maintenance dose necessary to produce a therapeutic serum level may be

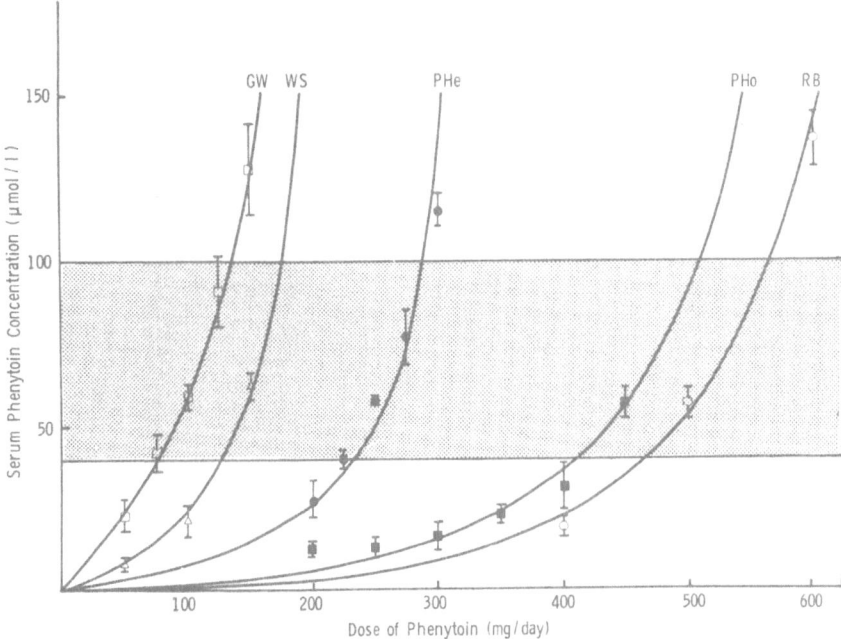

Figure 2. Relationship between daily maintenance dose and serum phenytoin concentration in five patients. Each point represents the mean (± SD) of 3–8 separate measurements of serum phenytoin concentration on a given dose of drug. Sufficient time was allowed between changes in dose for steady state to be achieved. The hatched area indicates a slightly more generous therapeutic range than is given in the text. The curves were fitted by computer, using the Michaelis-Menten equation (Richens and Dunlop 1975a).

made from a determination of the plasma half-life following a single dose. However, this may not be very practical on a routine basis, especially with drugs that have a long half-life as a several-day admission to hospital would be required for this to be carried out. For phenytoin, the process is even more complicated because of the saturable nature of its metabolism, and it is necessary to calculate K_m and V_{max} values rather than a half-life. Two methods have been suggested using two steady-state serum levels for the

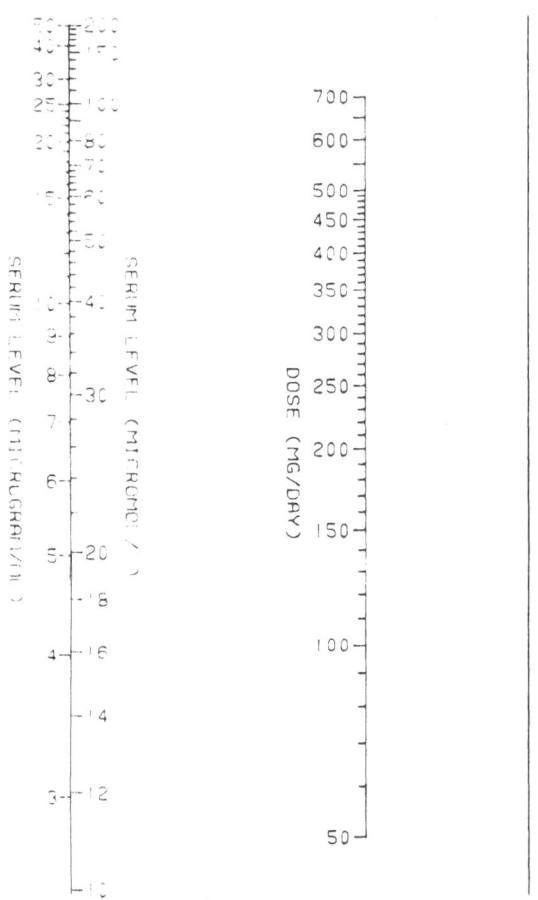

Figure 3. Nomogram for calculating increments in phenytoin dosage. Given a single reliable dose of phenytoin, the dose required to produce a desired serum level can be predicted. A line is drawn connecting the observed serum level (left-hand scale) with the dose administered (centre scale) and extended to intersect the right-hand vertical line. From the point of intersection, another line is drawn back to the desired serum level (left-hand scale) and the dose necessary to produce this level can be read off the centre scale. Note this nomogram will give misleading predictions if the serum level measurement is inaccurate, if the patient's compliance is in doubt, if a change in concurrent treatment has been made since the starting level was measured, or if the phenytoin preparation is changed.

calculation (Ludden et al. 1976; Mullen 1977). A simpler nomogram approach requiring only one steady-state level has been proposed (Richens and Dunlop 1975b) and a revised version of the nomogram is illustrated in fig. 3 (Rambeck et al. 1978). This method on average produces good predictions (fig. 4), but its weakness is that it assumes that K_m does not vary from one patient to another – see Richens (1978) for discussion. Probably none of these methods will replace simply giving a dose, monitoring the serum level, and adjusting the dose in appropriate increments until a therapeutic level is obtained.

It is essential that the clinician responsible for drug prescribing can interpret the laboratory result correctly and is aware of the pitfalls which stand in his way. All laboratory tests get abused, and drug levels are no exception. One of the dangers is that the clinician concentrates too hard on the serum level and forgets to look at the patient–pharmacokinetically the treatment may be impeccable but lack of response to the drug chosen will only be detected by good clinical observation, not by serum levels. The latter provide only additional information which should be taken along with all the other clinical and laboratory evidence.

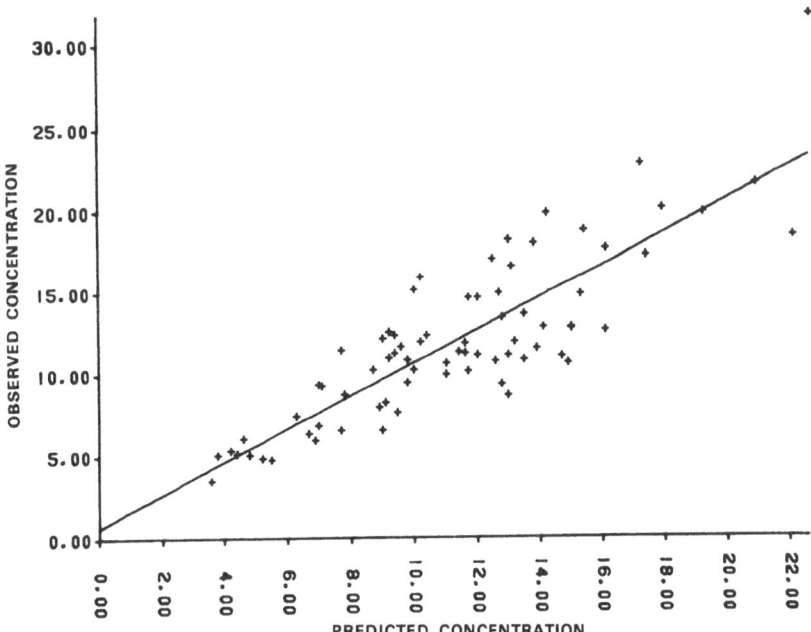

Figure 4. Correlation between observed serum level and the level predicted by use of the nomogram (fig. 3) following a change of phenytoin dose in 75 epileptic patients (Rambeck et al. 1978). The concentration axes are in mg/l (note: 1 mg/l $= 4 \mu$mol/l). Slope: 1.004 (not significantly different from 1); intersect: 0.67 (not significantly different from 0); r: 0.847 ($t = 13.6, p < 0.001$).

Herein lies the danger of therapeutic ranges of serum levels. Some excellent work has been performed, particularly by Lund (1974), in defining the therapeutic range for phenytoin, namely 40–80 μmol/l (10–20 mg/l). Although it is true that most patients appear to respond best when the level is within this range, mild epilepsy may be completely controlled with a "sub-therapeutic" level, while severe epilepsy may be little influenced even with a level in the toxic range. Adjusting the dose to produce a level within the range of 40–80 μmol/l may not always be in the patient's interest. Nevertheless, therapeutic ranges are a useful guide, and we need more prospective studies to define the ranges of some of the other drugs. Apart from phenytoin, ethosuximide is the only other antiepileptic drug whose therapeutic range has been clearly defined (Browne et al. 1975). For some drugs, the therapeutic ranges often quoted are meaningless: primidone, for example, has not yet been shown to be anticonvulsant in its parent form in man, and therefore it is misleading to quote a therapeutic range for it.

One occasional, but particularly valuable, contribution of serum level monitoring is in recognizing masked drug intoxication. While phenytoin intoxication is usually immediately recognizable from the characteristic triad of coarse nystagmus, ataxia and slurred speech, occasionally the presentation is bizarre. Choreo-athetoid movements may occur in the absence of the classical toxic signs, and degenerative disorders, dementia, psychosis, and cerebral tumour may be simulated. For instance, I recently saw a fifty-year-old woman who had been rescued from a geriatric unit where she had been placed with a diagnosis of presenile dementia; in fact, she had a phenytoin level of 180 μmol/l and following a drug reduction her dementia and involuntary movements rapidly regressed. Sometimes a paradoxical increase in fit frequency can occur with intoxication and this may be mistaken for under-treatment. It is important, therefore, that serum levels are monitored if any odd neuropsychiatric disturbance occurs in an epileptic patient.

One important advance to come from our ability to monitor serum drug levels has been our greater understanding of the kinetic behaviour of drugs in the body. The extent and predictability of absorption of oral preparations can be studied and improved, and a knowledge of the elimination half-life has allowed us to make more logical recommendations concerning the dose interval. For example, it has been traditional to give phenytoin and phenobarbitone three times daily, but it is now known that both of these compounds have half-lives compatible with once daily administration, both in adults and children (Cocks et al. 1975). Phenytoin is an interesting example in this context because the usually quoted values for its plasma half-life, e.g. 22 hours (Arnold and Gerber 1970), grossly overestimate its rate of metabolism when a therapeutic serum level is achieved. It has been shown (Richens 1975b) that the *effective* half-life of the drug lengthens as the serum concentration rises (it might be less confusing to say that the clearance of the drug diminishes as the concentration rises) and therefore the fluctuation in serum level becomes relatively smaller at higher concentrations (fig. 5). This is one benefit that is derived from phenytoin's saturable kinetics, although in other respects this property is a disadvantage.

Phenytoin is very badly absorbed from intramuscular sites of injection, although this was not recognized until it was possible to measure serum levels (Wilensky and Lowden 1973). The drug is relatively insoluble and therefore in order to dissolve 250 mg in an acceptable volume of solution, organic solvents have to be used and the pH of the solution has to be adjusted to around 12. Following injection into a muscle, the solution is buffered to physiological pH and the drug crystallizes out and the crystals so formed present a small surface area for redissolution. Up to half of the drug may still be present in the muscle twenty-four hours after injection. Phenytoin should therefore never be given intramuscularly for status epilepticus, and it is probably better to avoid this route altogether. If parenteral administration is necessary, it can be given slowly intravenously once a day.

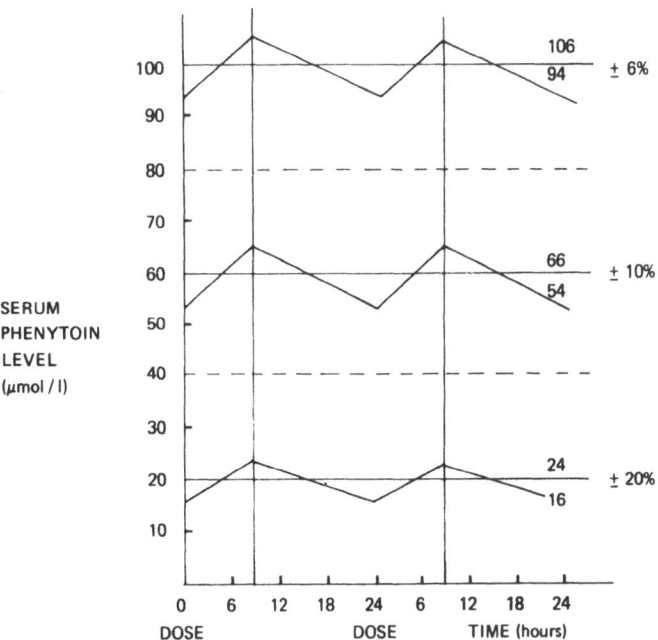

Figure 5. A theoretical plot of the fluctuation in serum level with once daily phenytoin dosing in an average patient with a subtherapeutic level (bottom), a therapeutic level (middle), and a toxic level (top). The plot was constructed using half-life data derived from Richens (1975b). The horizontal line drawn through each plot represents the mean level. Peak and trough concentrations and the percentage fluctuation in serum level are given on the right. The dashed lines indicate the therapeutic range of serum concentrations.

Monitoring serum drug levels has also led to a rapid advance in our understanding of drug interactions (Richens 1975b) and these are so common with phenytoin that it is wise to monitor the serum level if another drug is added to or withdrawn from existing therapy.

A further benefit of drug monitoring is that compliance is improved, probably for two reasons. First, the patient is more likely to take his tablets if he knows that his omission is going to be detected at his next visit to the clinic, and second, the results can be discussed with the patient and provide an opportunity for better communication, lack of which is a major factor in producing non-compliance.

Table 1 summarizes the indications for measuring serum phenytoin levels, as well as some of the circumstances in which drug levels should not be measured.

QUALITY CONTROL

The last topic that I would like to touch upon is that of quality control. I have now had six years experience in organizing an international quality control scheme for antiepileptic drug assays (Richens, 1975a, 1978a, 1978b) which was begun because my early experience in measuring phenytoin levels made me aware that there was considerable inter-laboratory variation in these assays. Nowhere has this been better illustrated than in the blind survey organized by Pippenger et al. (1976) in which aliquots of pooled sera containing phenytoin, phenobarbitone, primidone and ethosuximide were mailed to a large number of North American laboratories. For each specimen

Table 1. Indications regarding measurement of serum phenytoin levels.

Indications for measuring phenytoin levels:
1. Seizures not controlled by average or high doses of the drug
2. Increase in seizure frequency in a previously well stabilized patient
3. If intoxication is suspected
4. If odd neuropsychiatric symptoms occur
5. Before addition or removal of another drug
6. Suspected non-compliance
7. Status epilepticus occurring in a patient receiving phenytoin
8. Epilepsy in childhood, when pharmacokinetic variation is much greater

Contra-indications for measuring serum drug levels:
1. When therapeutic range of serum levels is not known because of
   (a) doubtful efficacy or (b) insufficient research
2. Seizures well controlled by an average dose of drug

Abuse of drug assays:
1. In order to delay making a decision about a patient – hoping the problem will go away
2. Treating the serum level rather than the patient

```
SAMPLE: TEST SERUM L
DRUG: PHENYTOIN


DRUG      NO
LEVEL


          * * * * * * * * * * * * * * * * * * * * * * * * * * * * * *
20.00     0 *                                                       *
22.33     J *                                                       *
24.67     0 *                                                       *
27.00     J *                                                       *
29.33     0 *                                                       *
31.67     1 * X                                                     *
34.00     J *                                                       *
36.33     0 *                                                       *
38.67     1 * X                                                     *
41.00   - 4-*-X X X X X - - - - - - - - - - - - - - - - - - - - - -*
43.33     1 * X                                                     *
45.67     5 * X X X X X X                                           *
48.00     5 * X X X X X X                                           *
50.33    12 * X X X X X X X X X X X X X X                           *
52.67    10 * X X X X X X X X X X X                                 *
55.00    20 * X X X X X X X X X X X X X X X X X X X X X X X X        *
57.33    22 * X X X X X X X X X X X X X X X X X X X X X X X X X X X  *
59.67     8 * X X X X X X X X X X                                   *
62.00     7 * X X X X X X X X X                                     *
64.33     3 * X X X X                                               *
66.67     5 * X X X X X X                                           *
69.00     1 * X                                                     *
71.33     0 *                                                       *
73.67     2 * X X                                                   *
76.00     1 * X                                                     *
78.33     0 *                                                       *
80.67   - U-*- - - - - - - - - - - - - - - - - - - - - - - - - - -*
83.00     J *                                                       *
85.33     J *                                                       *
87.67     U *                                                       *
          * * * * * * * * * * * * * * * * * * * * * * * * * * * * * *


NUMBER ACCEPTED          107
NUMBER REJECTED            4
MEAN                   56.58
STANDARD DEVIATION      6.92
COEF OF VARIATION      12.23%
MINIMUM                39.30
MAXIMUM                77.80
MEDIAN                 56.81
MODE                   58.50
SPIKED VALUE           57.40
```

Figure 6. A good set of results obtained in the St. Bartholomew's Hospital Quality Control Scheme for Antiepileptic Drugs. The 111 laboratories measured the phenytoin concentration in a specimen of calf serum spiked with eight antiepileptic drugs. An individualized copy of this computer write-out is mailed to all participants. Results are in μmol/l, and the therapeutic range of serum concentrations (40–80 μmol/l) is indicated by the dashed lines. The mean value of 56.58 μmol/l was close to the spiked value of 57.40 μmol/l, and the coefficient of variation (12.23 percent) was one of the best results to date. However, of the four results rejected, three fell outside the range of the histogram; these results were 15.9, 95.0 and 99.0 μmol/l. On this specimen, therefore, which contained a therapeutic concentration of phenytoin, three results were in the subtherapeutic range and two were toxic.

the range of results reported was from zero to toxic, and coefficients of variation were from 38 to 505 percent. Following these alarming findings, Dr. Charles Pippenger set up a North American quality control scheme, while the programme that I initiated grew into a scheme, the St. Bartholomew's Hospital Quality Control Scheme for Antiepileptic Drugs, which currently includes 204 laboratories in most Western European countries and in South Africa, Malaysia and Australia.

Although our coefficients of variation are usually much smaller (e.g. fig. 6) than those found by Pippenger et al. they are still large enough for us to be able to say that good internal and external quality control is absolutely essential if the clinician is to have confidence in the assay results produced by a laboratory. This is, of course, long-accepted practice in clinical chemistry. In drug measurement, however, it is even more important because (1) drugs are generally more difficult to estimate; (2) interference from other drugs is common unless highly specific techniques are used; and (3) there is no "normal range" to alert to the possibility of a methodological error. Anti-epileptic drugs are mostly present in high concentrations in serum and therefore the analytical problems with these compounds are smaller than we will face when our attention is turned to drugs which, weight for weight, are much more potent than the antiepileptic drugs. Perhaps our assay methods will keep pace with our needs (e.g. immunoassay), but if the reputation of the drug monitoring laboratory is to be established and maintained, we will have to give priority to quality control, and this means not only running internal quality control specimens with routine assays, but also checking our results against other laboratories on an external scheme. In order to provide the latter in areas other than antiepileptic drugs, the St. Bartholomew's Hospital scheme is being extended to encompass tricyclic antidepressants and theophylline.

REFERENCES

Arnold, K. and Gerber, N., The rate of decline of diphenylhydantoin in human plasma. *Clinical Pharmacology and Therapeutics* 11, 121–134 (1970).
Browne, T.R., Dreifuss, F.E., Dyken, P.R., Goode, D.J., Penry, J.K., Porter, R.J. and White, P.T., Ethosuximide in the treatment of absence (petit mal) seizures. *Neurology* 25, 515–524 (1975). Minneapolis.
Cocks, D.A., Critchley, E.M.R., Hayward, H.W., Owen, V., Mawer, G.E. and Woodcock, B.G., Control of epilepsy with a single daily dose of phenytoin sodium. *British Journal of Clinical Pharmacology* 2, 449–453 (1975).
Koch-Weser, J., The serum level approach to individualization of drug dosage. *European Journal of Clinical Pharmacology* 9, 1–8 (1975).
Ludden, T.M., Allen, J.P., Valutsky, W.A., Vicuna, A.V., Napp, J.M., Hoffman, S.F., Wallace, J.F., Lalka, D. and McNay, J.L., Individualization of phenytoin dosage regimens. *Clinical Pharmacology and Therapeutics* 21, 287–293 (1976).
Lund, L., Anticonvulsant effects of diphenylhydantoin relative to plasma levels: a prospective 3 year study in ambulant seizures. *Archives of Neurology* 31, 289–294 (1974). Chicago.

Mullen, P.W., A novel graphical procedure for individualizing phenytoin therapy. *British Journal of Clinical Pharmacology* 4, 733P–734P (1977).

Pippenger, C.E., Penry, J.K., White, B.G., Daly, D.D. and Buddington, R., Interlaboratory variability in determination of plasma antiepileptic drug concentrations. *Archives of Neurology* 33, 351–355 (1976). Chicago.

Rambeck, B., Boenick, H. E., Dunlop, A. and Richens, A., Predicting phenytoin dose. A revised nomogram. Therapeutic Drug Monitoring (in press).

Reynolds, E.H., Chadwick, D. and Galbraith, A.W., One drug (phenytoin) in the treatment of epilepsy. *Lancet* 1, 923–926 (1976).

Richens, A., Reuslts of a phenytoin quality control scheme. In: *Clinical Pharmacology of Anti-Epileptic Drugs*. Ed., Schneider, H., et al., Heidelberg, 1975a.

Richens, A., A Study of the pharmacokinetics of phenytoin (diphenylhydantoin) in epileptic patients, and the development of a nomogram for making dose increments. *Epilepsia* 16, 627–647 (1975b).

Richens, A., Interactions with antiepileptic drugs. *Drugs* 13, 266–275 (1977).

Richens, A., Antiepileptic drugs. In: *Recent Advances in Clinical Pharmacology*, vol. 1. Ed., Shand, D. and Turner, P., Edinburgh, 1978.

Richens, A., Drug level monitoring – quantity and quality. *British Journal of Clinical Pharmacology* 5, 285–288 (1978a).

Richens, A., Anticonvulsant clinics. In: *Clinical Pharmacology and Patient Care*. Ed., Rawlins, M.D., London, 1978b.

Richens, A. and Dunlop, A., Serum phenytoin levels in the management of epilepsy. *Lancet* 2, 247–248 (1975a).

Richens, A. and Dunlop, A., Phenytoin dosage nomogram. *Lancet* 2, 1305–1306 (1975b).

Richens, A., Dunlop, A., Ahmad, S. and Laidlaw, J., Monitoring serum phenytoin. *Lancet* 1, 699–700 (1976).

Serrano, E.E. and Wilder, B.J., Intramuscular administration of diphenylhydantoin: histological follow-up. *Archives of Neurology* 31, 276–278 (1974). Chicago.

Shorvon, S.D. and Reynolds, E.H., Unnecessary polypharmacy for epilepsy. *British Medical Journal* 1, 1635–1637 (1977).

Shorvon, S.D., Chadwick, D., Galbraith, A.W. and Reynolds, E.H., One drug for epilepsy. *British Medical Journal* 1, 474–476 (1978).

Wilensky, A.J. and Lowden, J.A., Inadequate serum levels after intramuscular administration of diphenylhydantoin. *Neurology* 23, 318–324 (1973) Minneapolis.

PART IIA

APPLICATIONS TO SPECIFIC DRUGS

5. ANTIEPILEPTIC DRUGS

E. VAN DER KLEIJN AND T.B. VREE

Drugs, here defined as substances that are body-foreign by nature or amount, often initiate a sequence of biochemical and physiological processes. Body-foreign substances, semantically distinguished as food, luxury, or drug are absorbed, distributed in and eliminated from tissues and organs in either intact or modified form by a multitude of mechanisms. The rates at which these processes occur simultaneously are characteristic for every drug with the restrictions of a number of variables. These rates determine the onset, the time course, and the intensity of beneficial or toxic effect to the body.

Pharmacokinetics involves the studies of these rates of absorption from the various loci of administration, of distribution in the body, of metabolic transformation and of elimination. The application of the information obtained from theoretical and experimental pharmacokinetics for the treatment of patients is further specified by the adjective *clinical*.

It is the aim of clinical pharmacokinetics to describe the relation between the dose administered to an individual patient, and the concentration that results in blood, plasma or any other body fluid available for sampling, in organs and in tissues and if possible in the so-called bio-phase near or on the receptors, as a variable of time. It tries by measurements of pharmacodynamic parameters to link these results with the beneficial or adverse results of the administration of the drug. This chapter deals with a number of conditions and variables that can influence the value and reliability of the pharmacokinetic parameters of some antiepileptic drugs that can analytically be assayed in clinical conditions.

In patients one is bound to practical limitations, e.g., the number of samples and dosage schedules used in individuals. This does not allow the estimation of all possible parameters like time-constant or biological half-life, apparent volume of distribution, etc., but does allow calculation of the clearance. The value of clearance parameters for patient treatment will be discussed.

PHARMACOKINETIC REASONING

In abstract pharmacokinetic terms it can be expressed that amounts of drug are homogeneously distributed in compartments of particular volumes.

The resulting concentrations are subject to continuous change as a result of input and output of the materials. The dominant driving forces are hemodynamics, secretion and enzyme-substrate reactions. In treatment with drugs the compound can mathematically be considered distributed in a single compartment (van der Kleijn et al. 1972, 1975). This model appears to be justified even though distribution studies have revealed selective accumulation of drug in body regions generally not accessible for sampling. For these drugs, with the exception of phenytoin, salicylic acid, barbiturates in toxic overdosages, and 4-hydroxybutyrate, the conditions of linear proportionality between amount of drug administered and concentration in the plasma and body regions is reasonably fulfilled.

The exceptions show a non-linear relationship due to enzyme capacity limited elimination. When the rate of elimination (k_{el}) is small (half-life is large) and the time interval between two dosages (Δt) is small, chronic intermittent (oral) drug administration can be considered to correspond to continuous linear infusion. In clinical practice one will not allow oscillations in amount or in concentration of more than ten to twenty percent. Considering a simple one-compartment distribution model, the biological half-life ($t_{1/2}$) of the drug has to account for more than 6.6 or 3.1 respectively times the dosage interval. When $t_{1/2}$ appears to be shorter one has to consider:

1. Decreasing the dosage interval (Δt);
2. Choosing a "pro" or "precursor" drug or a formulation with sustained release;
3. Infusing the drug intravenously;
4. Allowing fluctuations of more than twenty percent.

Although more complicated models may sometimes be more justified, simple one-compartment distribution kinetics can often satisfactorily serve the clinical purpose. In *epilepsy* one tries to maintain about 21 mg of phenobarbital per kg body weight and for phenytoin the amount accounts for about 8.4 mg/kg. Of these amounts about 14 percent of phenobarbital and 60 percent of phenytoin are eliminated daily and need to be compensated by the dose at the appropriate frequency. This means that 3 mg/kg of phenobarbital and 5.2 mg/kg of phenytoin have to be administered every twenty-four hours. The frequency or the administration interval (Δt interval = 1 : frequency) needs to be adapted so that the oscillations in amount remain within the therapeutic limits. Every substance therefore needs its own frequency. For the mathematical expressions and interpretation of pharmacokinetic models one is referred to the extensive literature on this matter (van der Kleijn et al. 1975; Wagner 1973). In clinical practice of chronic intermittent oral treatment, the following equations can be applied:

$$C_{\text{therap}} = \text{dose}/(k_{el} \times V_d \times \Delta t) \tag{1}$$

$$C_{\text{therap}} = \text{dose}/(\dot{V}_{\text{el}} \times \Delta t) \qquad (2)$$

$$C_{\text{therap}} = \text{dose} \times t_{1/2}/(0.69 \times V_d \times \Delta t) \qquad (3)$$

In these equations V_{el}^* is the elimination clearance (1/h); V_d is the apparent volume of distribution (1); k_{el} is the rate constant for elimination (1/h). When a reliable statistical correlation has been found with body weight the equation can be written as

$$C_{\text{therap}} = \text{dose}/(\dot{V}_{\text{el}}' \times \Delta t \times W) \qquad (4)$$

in which $\dot{V}_{\text{el}}'$ is the relative clearance per kg body weight (W); C_{therap} is the plasma concentration relevant for the control of a particular degree of the disease. The term relative clearance has been chosen so far in an adult patient population since a linear correlation with body weight has been found for a number of drugs. This, however, remains an arbitrary reference. Sometimes a better value is obtained when $\dot{V}_{\text{el}}$ is related to body surface (fig. 1). The bioavailability factor F is always considered to be 1 or is included in the $\dot{V}_{\text{el}}'$ value otherwise (table 1).

However, there are more variables that have to be taken into account when considering clearance values. For phenytoin the relation between dose per time and concentration has been shown to be non-linear (Richens

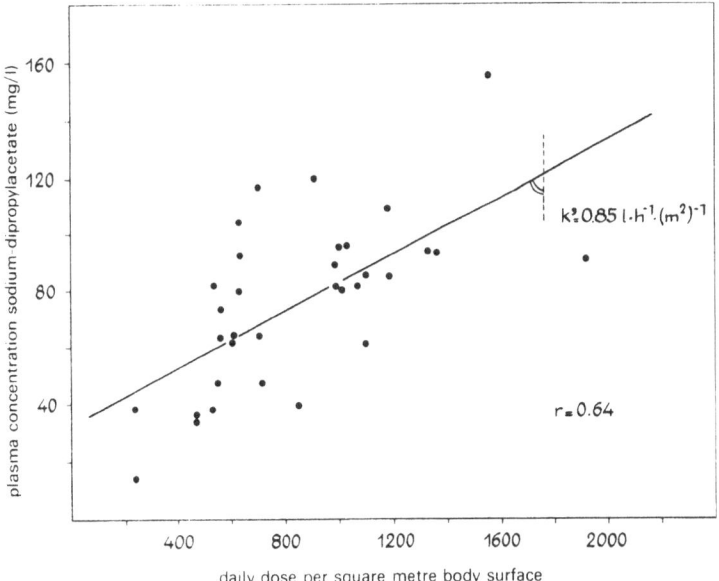

Figure 1. Absence of confident linearity between the dose administered and the resulting plasma concentration of Valproate (dipropylacetate) in epileptic patients. The $\dot{V}_{\text{el}}/m^2$ body surface, although poor, appeared to give a more confident correlation than per kg body weight.

Table 1. Mean values of pharmacokinetic parameters.

Drug	V'_{el} (l/h·kg)	C_{therap} (mg/l)	Δt (h)	C_{tox} (mg/l)	$t_{1/2}$ (h)	V' (l/kg)	Time to reach C_{therap} (days)	t_{max} (h)
Phenobarbital	0.005	30–40	12	100	120–150	0.7	25	2–4
Phenytoin	0.020	12–15	8	20	10–100[a]	0.7	3	2–4
Primidone[b]	0.060	8–10	8	15	6–10	1	1.5	1–3
Ethosuximide	0.018	60–80	8	150	30–40	0.65	6	1–3
Sodium valproate	0.012	60–80	6	200	7–10	0.25	1.5	1–2
Carbamazepine	0.030–0.150	5–8	8	25	35[c]	2	4	6–12
Clonazepam	0.100–0.250	0.03–0.06	8	0.1	30	3.3	5	3–4
Diazepam[d]	0.030	0.4–0.6	8	1	32	1.8	5	3–4
Nitrazepam	0.075	0.08–0.12	8	0.2	20	1.8	3	2–4

The mean values have generally been obtained from statistical studies (Guelen et al. 1975) or from literature data. When combinations need to be prescribed the values may have to be adapted, e.g., according to table 2.

a Non-linear kinetics possible. Phenytoin (non-linear parameters) K_m = 4–15mg/l, V_{max} = 0.4–0.7 mg/l.h.

b Primidone is metabolized to phenobarbital and phenylethyl malonylurea (PEMA) with their own antiepileptic activity.

c Half-life decreases during chronic treatment to approximately 10–15 hours; V'_{el} increases therefore three to four times.

d Diazepam is metabolized to desmethyldiazepam with its own antiepileptic activity.

1975). Non-linear or enzyme capacity limited elimination with $K_m = 4$–15 mg/l will show its influence in the therapeutic concentration range of phenytoin of 12–15 mg/l. This phenomenon can be expressed mathematically for clinical application by the equation in which the reciprocal time is constant and thus clearance has become concentration-dependent (fig. 2):

$$C = \text{dose } (V'_{el} \times \Delta t \times W) \tag{5}$$

or

$$C = \frac{\text{dose} \cdot K_m}{\Delta t \times V_{max} \times V' \times W \times - \text{dose}} \tag{6}$$

in which K_m is the apparent Michaelis-Menten constant (mg/l) and V_{max} the apparent maximum rate of metabolism (mg.h^{-1})

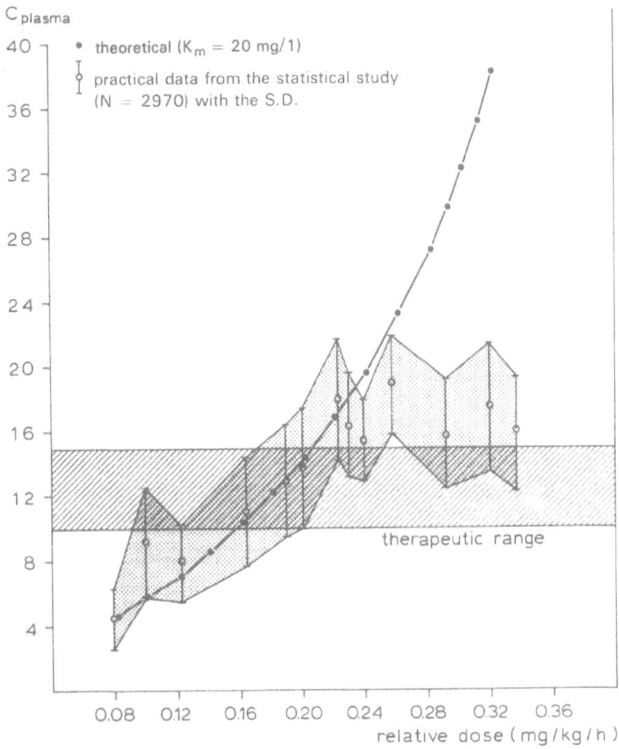

Figure 2. Theoretical relationship between dose of phenytoin per day and resulting concentration in plasma according to equation 8. Patient data are included showing deviation of the theoretical relationship due to lack of patient compliance.

CALCULATION OF MAINTENANCE DOSAGE REGIMEN

The equation above can also be rearranged for the calculation of the individual dosage regimen in cases of exponential elimination processes:

$$\text{dose} = \dot{V}'_{el} \times C_{\text{therap}} \times \Delta_t \times W \tag{7}$$

When the clearance has become concentration-dependent, thus when metabolism appears to be enzyme capacity limited, the following equation can be applied:

$$\text{dose} = \frac{V_{\text{max}}}{K_m + C} \times V' \times C \times \Delta t \times W \tag{8}$$

Adequate and statistically confident K_m, V_{max} and V' data of drugs determined under clinical conditions of pathology, co-medication, and nutrition, among other variables, are not yet available for practical use with patients.

Non-linear binding characteristics at the tissue level can occur when linearity exists for plasma protein binding, especially when drugs have a large tissue-to-plasma partition coefficient. This may complicate the problem and needs intensive investigation.

When enough concentration time data are obtained for an individual, the Michaelis-Menten constant K_m, V_{max} and V' can be calculated by means of a numerical method (van Ginneken et al. 1974). A graphical method has been proposed by Ludden et al. (1976) by plotting plasma concentration values following dosage increments (fig. 3).

INTERPRETATION OF CLEARANCE PARAMETER IN CLINICAL PHARMACOKINETICS

Although the clearance can be considered as a constant the conditions for which the value applies have to be well defined. Clearance values can be determined under clinical conditions by using equation 7 (Guelen et al. 1975), deriving it from plasma concentration values determined in the laboratory and from the physician's therapeutic data, such as: dosage regimen-dose (D), time interval (Δt); and body weight and length (allowing the calculation and statistical analyses to body surface). With data on sex, age, concomitant drugs, nutrition (if abnormal), dosage form and brand, period of previous medication, sampling time, clinical pathology (e.g. renal function), it is possible to select statistically for best homogeneous population (Guelen et al. 1975) allowing the calculation of the most confident clearance value under the defined conditions.

The clearance value for a drug can also be derived from C_{ss}, dose per

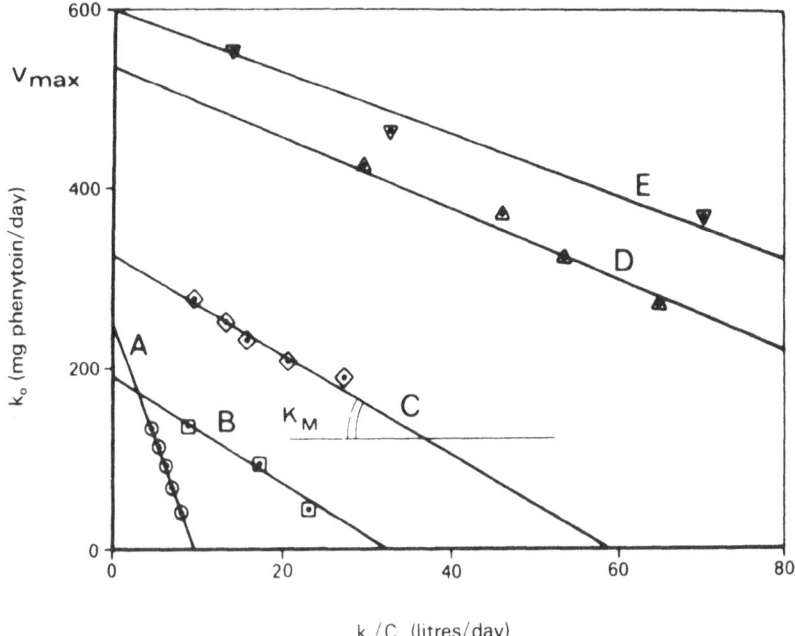

Figure 3. Graphical determination of apparent V_{max} and K_m value according to Ludden et al. (1976).

time per kg body weight graphs often found in the literature. From equation 2 (Guelen et al. 1975) it can be seen that the reciprocal of the slope of this linear regression line equals the relative clearance (fig. 1). The statistics of these regression lines supply the confidence parameter of this clearance value. Absence of linearity of this regression may also lead to identification of enzyme capacity limited elimination (fig. 2). Poor confidence will stimulate search for variables that may improve the homogeneity of the population. So far the following variables have been identified for a number of antiepileptic drugs (Guelen et al. 1975). An attempt has been made to quantitate them for practical use in patients.

1. Body weight or surface;
2. Age;
3. Sex;
4. Pathology, e.g. liver and kidney function, stress, and so on;
5. Absorption characteristics;
6. Co-medication;
7. Influence of aphysiological concentration of endogenous substance on tissue distribution, distribution volume, and other factors.

Comparison of results from routine plasma concentrations with these statistically obtained parameters also enables checks on laboratory performance and assay method. When these qualities are warranted by internal standardization and standard samples it may be possible that deviating clearance values help to identify, diagnose and evaluate:

A. Pathology;

B. Lack of patient adherence to the prescriber's regimen and total medication profile;

C. Erratic pharmacokinetics, e.g. non-linear kinetics, multi-compartment kinetics, absorption and elimination dysfunctions, first-pass metabolism;

D. Influence of co-medication or nutrition;

E. Quality of the formulation (limited bioavailability, e.g., for sustained release preparations);

F. Inadequate route of administration;

G. Instability of the sample.

Before a dosage regimen is corrected, it is advisable to consider and weigh these factors. When changes are made or observed a new sample should be analysed after more than five times the $t_{1/2}$ of the drug following the change, to check its influence on the normal value for these conditions. Next to the identification of the above factors plasma concentrations may support diagnosis of:

H. Toxic, adequate or subtherapeutic results in particular when clinical symptomatology does not permit distinguishability between states of over- or underdosing. For instance, antiepileptic drugs may be epileptogenic at high levels and benzodiazepines may elicit excitatory states. When not identified, these symptoms may lead to increase of the dose or the addition of a related compound that may result in serious problems.

When the diagnosis is clinically confirmed it may result in:

1. Correction of dosage regimen;
2. Treatment of the disease states;
3. Enforcement of the intake;
4. Addition or withdrawal of one or more drugs;
5. Change to another formulation or route of administration.

ESTABLISHMENT OF THERAPEUTICALLY RELEVANT PLASMA CONCENTRATION

The therapeutically relevant plasma concentration, C_{therap} has been determined for a number of drugs. These values have been evaluated from careful clinical studies by closely monitoring the predefined objective effects, adverse effects or lack of effect in relation to a confident plasma concentration profile. Due to the difficulties in medical semantics and the multitude of experimental variables in patients these values often show large variations.

Assuming reasonable control of the disease state in epilepsy institutions through the daily self-control or monitoring by the accompanying nurses and doctors, therapeutic optimum values can also be obtained from epidemiological studies on plasma concentrations in large populations. There is little information on the therapeutic concentration values when combinations of drugs are given. Moreover it has been observed in epilepsy that extremely low concentrations of either one or more drugs are reported to be effective. Withdrawal of the drug has been reported to precipitate crises. This paradoxical phenomenon also needs further confirmation and investigation. The quantitative dependency of C_{therap} on, for instance, severity of the disease state and also of technical factors like laboratory and assay quality, chemical stability of the sample and sampling time often still needs clarification through inter-laboratory controls and standards. Similar to what has been routine in clinical chemistry, standardization is necessary to compare the results of different laboratories, methods, chemists, times of the day, week or month. The usefulness and necessity of such quality control has been proven (Richens 1975).

TIME REQUIRED TO REACH THE STEADY-STATE CONCENTRATION

Although administration of rapid intravenous bolus injections may be indicated in acute critical conditions such as status epilepticus, for diazepam or clonazepam, and for acute digitalization it is impossible to reach equilibrium plateau concentrations throughout the body before a period of at least four to five times $t_{1/2}$ has elapsed and the drug has been given as sequential intermittent treatment or intravenous linear infusion (table 1). The same holds when a change in the dosage regimen has been made or when a change in one of the aforementioned conditions A–G has been established.

CALCULATION OF MAINTENANCE DOSAGE FOR COMBINATIONS OF DRUGS

The influence of drugs on the clearance of other drugs may require dose adaptations when C_{therap} has to be maintained. Both increase and decrease of the clearance as a result of co-medication have been reported. Decrease

Table 2. Correction factor (M) for the mean relative clearance value of antiepileptic drugs in combinations (Guelen et al. 1975).

Drug	$V_{el}^{*\prime}$(l/h.kg)	M	*In combination with*
Phenytoin	0.0199	1.00	
Phenytoin	0.0188	0.94	Phenobarbital
Phenytoin	0.0174	0.87	Carbamazepine
Phenytoin	0.0231	1.16	Primidone
Phenytoin	0.023	1.16	Phenobarbital and primidone
Phenytoin	0.016	0.80	Phenobarbital and carbamazepine
Phenytoin	0.018	0.90	Primidone and carbamazepine
Phenytoin	0.0165	0.83	Primidone, phenobarbital and carbamazepine
Carbamazepine	0.132	1.00	After chronic treatment
Carbamazepine	0.151	1.14	Phenobarbital
Carbamazepine	0.204	1.55	Phenytoin
Phenobarbital	0.0053	1.00	
Phenobarbital	0.0042	0.79	Phenytoin
Phenobarbital	0.0044	0.83	Carbamazepine

of statistical confidence of the clearance values is also possible. This may present problems with the interpretation of the therapeutic efficacy.

An attempt has been made to quantitate the influence of well-defined co-medications. This would then allow calculation of the dose using the following equation with the co-medication factor M from table 2:

$$\text{dose} = V_{el}^{\prime} \times M \times C_{therap} \times \Delta t \times W \tag{9}$$

The statistical significance of this factor M has not yet been established satisfactorily. Further research by Guelen is currently under way.

CALCULATION OF MAINTENANCE DOSE FOR CHILDREN

Children generally require a relatively larger maintenance dose per kg body weight or m² body surface because of a relatively larger clearance of drugs, net result of a larger relative apparent distribution volume and a larger reciprocal time constant for elimination, k_{el} (shorter $t_{1/2}$). The correction factor to the mean adult dosage for antiepileptic drugs generally does not obey the classical, growth statistics-based, Young rule: age/(age + 12) × 100 = percentage of the adult dose. It appears that the Augsberger rule (4 × age + 20 = percentage adult dose) generally better serves the aims – see fig. 4 (van der Kleijn et al. 1974). When medication with more than one drug is considered, the dosage regimen should be corrected to the specifications of the

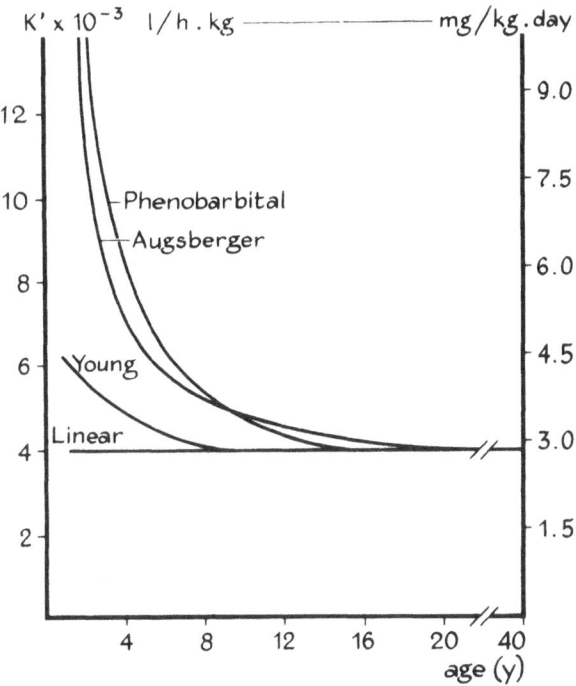

Figure 4. Relationship between clearance, age and required daily dose in patients treated only with phenobarbital. The relationship will differ statistically for patients treated with combinations of drugs. The equations of Young and of Augsberger have been translated to relative clearance by using table 3. The dosage required is calculated to reach a therapeutic plasma concentration of 30 mg phenobarbital per litre.

individual combination. The equation suitable for the calculation of children's dosages reads:

$$\text{child dose} = V'_{cl} \times A \times C_{\text{therap}} \times \Delta t \times W \tag{10}$$

in which A is the correction factor of the relative clearance for the given age of the patient (table 3), or

$$\text{child dose} = P \times \text{adult dose}/100 \tag{11}$$

in which P is the percentage of the dose of an adult (table 3). The mean Adult Dose will generally be found in regular textbooks.

CALCULATION OF STARTING DOSE

Due to the possible initial multi-compartment kinetics after a rapid bolus

Table 3. Percentage (*P*) of the adult dose for children and correction factor *A* for age of the relative clearance from table 1.

Age (years)	Denekamp (1962)	Young	Augsberger (1962)	Phenobarbital (Van der Kleijn et al. (1975)	
	P	P	P	P	A
0	11				
0.25	16				
0.5	19				
0.75	22.5				
1	24.5	7.7	24		
1.5	27.5				
2	30	14.3	28	35	3.50
3	34	20	32	40.5	2.70
4	38	25	36	43	2.15
5	42	29.5	40	45.5	1.82
6	44.5	33.3	44	48	1.60
7	48.5	36.8	48	50.7	1.45
8	52	40	52	52	1.30
9	55	45	56	56.3	1.25
10	60	50	60	59	1.18
11	64	55	64	59.4	1.08
12	69	60	68	63	1.05
13	75	65	72	66.7	1.02
14	81	70	76	70.7	1.01
15	84	75	80	75.8	1.01
16	90	80	84	80.5	1.006
17	95	85	88	85	1
18	100	90	92	90	1
19	100	100	100	95	1
20	100	100	100	100	1

injection V^1 may be smaller than V_{ss} after infusion. It may be possible to meet the therapeutic aim and the effective concentration in plasma by using the equation:

$$\text{dose} = C_{therap} \times V^1 \times W \tag{12}$$

or

$$\text{dose} = \frac{t_{1/2}}{0.69} \times V'_{cl} \times C_{therap} \times W \tag{13}$$

This dose is likely to produce initial side effects. When the clinical condition permits a more gentle start of the therapy it should be preferred to start with the maintenance dose and to wait for evaluation of the therapeutic effect until the time required to reach the steady-state concentration has passed, but an initial higher starting dosage regimen for a limited time period followed by continuation on an adapted maintenance regimen is often necessary.

CORRECTION OF THE DOSAGE REGIMEN WHEN INDIVIDUAL
CLEARANCE APPEARS TO MEET THE STATISTICAL NORMAL
VALUE AND THE THERAPEUTICALLY RELEVANT PLASMA
CONCENTRATION HAS NOT BEEN REACHED

When the intended plasma concentration (C_{therap}) and the clinically intended
effect has not been reached and the calculated clearance for the individual
appears to match the normal clearance value the dose can proportionally
be corrected:

$$\text{new dose} = \frac{\text{previous dose} \times C_{therap}}{C_{prev}} \tag{14}$$

Drugs that show enzyme capacity limited elimination, like phenytoin, will
need a more complicated non-linear correction taking into account the
K_m value:

$$\text{new dose} = \frac{(K_m + C_{prev}) \times C_{therap}}{(K_m + C_{therap}) \times C_{prev}} \times \text{previous dose} \tag{15}$$

Most of these parameters have to be reaffirmed in clinical conditions and
the validity and relevance has to be confirmed by further research. When
the metabolic parameters, e.g. K_m, are not available the correction can best
be achieved by careful monitoring of successive concentration assays upon
dosage increments.

$$K_m = \frac{D_2 \cdot C_1 \cdot C_2 - D_1 \cdot C_1 \cdot C_2}{D_1 \cdot C_2 - D_2 \cdot C_1} \tag{16}$$

Dose correction can also be achieved during this type of therapy by:

$$D_t = \frac{D_1 \cdot C_2 (C_2 - C_1)}{D_1 \cdot C_2 (C_t - C_1) - D_2 \cdot C_1 (C_t - C_2)} \cdot \frac{C_t}{C_2} \cdot D_2 \tag{17}$$

In these equations D_1 is the initially instituted dose at the chosen interval,
D_2 the newly chosen dose at the same interval, and C_1 and C_2 the measured
concentration values after the pseudo-steady state has been allowed to be
established (often five times $t_{1/2}$). C_t is the generally accepted therapeutic
concentration. Now the "therapeutic dose" (D_t) can be calculated. When
the calculated clearance of the individual does not meet the "normal" value
the aforementioned conditions A–G should be carefully checked and a new
sample should be analyzed. When a change in conditions has occurred,
one should wait until a new steady state is reached (table 1) before a new
sample is taken.

TIME INTERVAL OF DRUG ADMINISTRATION

To mimic the conditions of continuous infusion, thus minimizing fluctuations in plasma concentrations and effect, the dosage interval should be maintained as constant as possible. Although this creates many domestic problems it should be realized that the preferred schedules for drug administration in hospitals can be given as in table 4. The interval should be adapted to the specification of minimum fluctuations, e.g. ten to twenty percent. This may require a different interval for each drug depending on its $t_{1/2}$. The dosage interval can be calculated by the following hand rule:

$$\Delta t = t_{max} + t_{0.9} = t_{max} + 0.15 \cdot t_{1/2} \tag{18}$$

or

$$\Delta t = t_{max} + t_{0.8} = t_{max} + 0.32 \cdot t_{1/2} \tag{19}$$

in which t_{max} is the time to reach the maximum of absorption and $t_{0.9}$ and $t_{0.8}$ are the times in which the concentration has been reduced to ninety or eighty percent of its original value (table 1) respectively. It has been realized that in community practice, due to the problems of migration, complexity of working schedules, and so on, it is difficult to cope with such a regimen. The habit of prescribing too many drugs to be taken too frequently may lead to problems of patients compliance with their prescribed regimen. Unit dose distribution system and motivation and instruction have been experienced as improvements. Sustained release preparations and drugs with prolonged half-lives are worth developing as long as the total bioavailability of the drug will not be reduced.

PLASMA CONCENTRATION DETERMINATION

To attribute confident meaning to a plasma concentration value and the derived clearance parameter the sampling has to be carried out at such a time after the preceding drug administration that variation in time causes minimum variation in plasma and tissue concentration. As a result of the

Table 4. Preferred schedules for drug administration in hospitals.

Dosage frequency (per day)	Dosage interval (Δt)	Administration times
4	6	6.00, 12.00, 18.00, 0.00
3	8	6.00, 14.00, 22.00
2	12	6.00, 18.00
1	24	18.00

differences in kinetics of absorption, distribution and elimination of the different drugs these periods differ (table 5). The plasma specimen should be adequately stored to prevent decomposition; the time to process the sample should be short enough to have the patient benefit from the results (van der Kleijn et al. 1974). The accompanying request should mention at least civil data, body weight and length, drugs to be analysed, previous regimens, other drugs not to be analyzed, diet (if relevant), special instructions for use, and so on. When these data are not available plasma analyses can often be of little or no value. For the evaluation of the therapeutically relevant concentration and the calculated relative clearance, clinical chemistry data are of great importance.

SAMPLE MATERIAL

Kinetic parameters are usually based on plasma concentration determinations. When, however, invasive and painful blood sampling is not possible, it might be wise to make use of saliva. Next to that cerebrospinal fluid, tears, urine and wound exudates are sometimes available. When the total plasma concentration is measured the protein concentration may play a considerable role, because the pharmacological activity is supposed to be determined by the free concentration. The protein-binding capacity is of great importance for psychotropic drugs. In general because of their often high lipophilicity they show a high binding affinity for plasma protein.

Table 5. Antiepileptic drugs currently used and assayed for the clinical monitoring of patients.

Generic name	Sample time during chronic treatment (hours after intake)	Route	Sample volume (ml blood)	Assay method
Phenobarbital	4–12 protocol	oral intravenous	0.5–2	GC or EMIT
Phenytoin	4 protocol	oral intravenous	0.5–2	GC + methyl. or EMIT
Primidone	2–4	oral	0.5–2	GC + methyl. or EMIT
Ethosuximide	4	oral	0.5–1	GC
Valproate	2 and 6	oral	0.5–1	GC
Carbamazepine	4	oral	1–2	HPLC
Clonazepam	4	oral	2	GC + hydrol.
Diazepam	4 protocol	oral intravenous	2	GC
Nitrazepam	4	oral	2	HPLC

GC = gas chromatography; + methyl. = GC with flash methylation; + hydrol. = GC after hydrolysis; HPLC = high pressure liquid chromatography; EMIT = enzyme multiplied immunoassay technique; protocol = requires frequent sampling, e.g., at 0.5–1 h intervals.

Therefore in some cases it is necessary to take the albumin concentration of the sample material into account.

In this respect saliva might be a better reference for the free fraction (fig. 5). For acidic and amphoteric drugs this supposition seems to be reasonable. In table 6 the relationship of the concentration of antiepileptic drugs in saliva, cerebrospinal fluid (CSF) and serum are given. Saliva sampling appears to be attractive when a large number of samples is indicated in cases of "profile" determination. However, care should be taken for proper collection since the variation may depend on the moment of sampling in relation to intake of food and beverages. There may also be a difference in the excretes of parotic and submandibular glands.

Table 6. Relationship of the concentration of antiepileptic drugs in saliva, CSF and serum.

Drug	Ratio CSF/serum	Ratio saliva/serum ·
Phenobarbital	0.48	0.32
Phenytoin	0.11	0.10
Primidone	0.72	0.97
Carbamazepine	0.25	0.24
Valproate	0.10	0.06
Ethosuximide	0.92	0.88

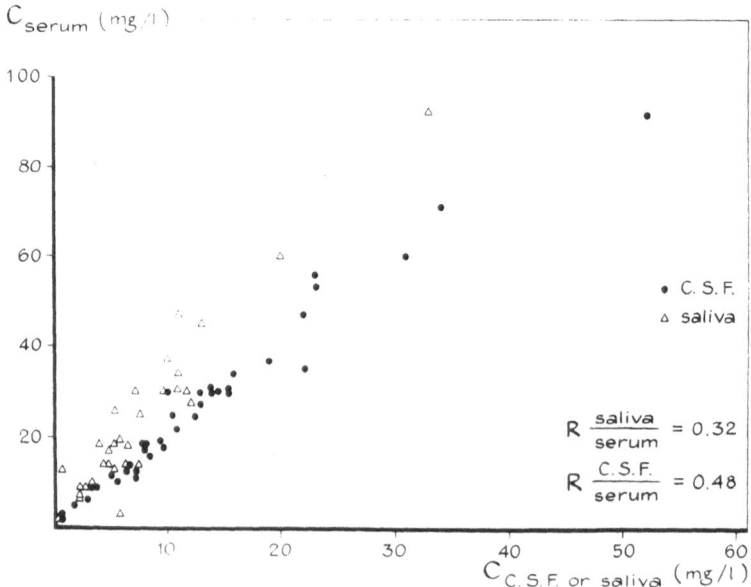

Figure 5. Relationship between the concentrations of phenobarbital measured in serum and saliva or cerebrospinal fluid (C.S.F.).

REFERENCES

Augsberger, A., Alte und neue Faustregeln für die Arzneidosierung bei Kindern. *Triangle* 5, 200 (1962).

Denekamp, A.E., Dosering van geneesmiddelen bij kinderen. *Huisarts en Wetensch* 5, 357 (1962).

Van Ginneken, C.A.M., van Rossum, J.M. and Fleuren, H.L.J.M., Linear and non-linear kinetics of drug elimination. *J. Pharmacokin. Biopharm* 2, 395–416 (1974).

Guelen, P.J.M., van der Kleijn, E. and Woudstra, U., Statistical evaluation of pharmacokinetic parameters of anti-epileptic drugs. In: *Clinical Pharmacology of Anti-Epileptic Drugs*. Ed., Schneider, H., et al. Heidelberg, 1975.

Van der Kleijn, E., Guelen, P.J.M., Baars, A.M., Vree, T.B., and Termond, E., The clearance and plasma concentration of antiepileptic and cardiac drugs as references for the calculation and individual monitoring of dosage regimens. *Pharm. Weekblad* 110, 49, 1222–1232 (1975).

Van der Kleijn, E., Guelen, P.J.M., van Wijk, C.G.W.M., Baars, I. and Vree, T.B., Clinical pharmacokinetics, a symposium. ed., Levy, G. *Am. Pharm. Assoc. Acad. Pharm. Sci.* 79–101 (1974).

Van der Kleijn, E., van Rossum, J.M., Muskens, E.T.J.M. and Rijntjes, N.V.M., Pharmacokinetics of diazepam in dogs. mice and humans, *Acta Pharmacolog.* 29, Suppl. 3, 109–127 (1972).

Van der Kleijn, E., Vree, T.B. and Guelen, P.J.M., Klinische farmacokinetiek van psychopharmaca. *Bulletin van de Coördinatiecommissie Biochemisch Onderzoek van de Sectie Psychiatrische Instituten van de Nationale Ziekenhuisraad* 76–3 (December), 46–68 (1976).

Ludden, F.M., Hawkins, D.W., Allen, J.P. and Hoffman, S.F., Optimum phenytoin dosage regimen. *Lancet* 307–308 (1976).

Richens, A., A study of the pharmacokinetics of phenytoin (diphenylhydantoin) in epileptic patients, and the development of a nomogram for making dose increments. *Epilepsia* 16, 627–647 (1975).

Wagner, J.G., Properties of the Michaëlis-Menten equation and its integrated form, which are useful in pharmacokinetics. *J. Pharmacokin. Biopharm* 1, 103–121 and 338 (1973).

6. LITHIUM

Long-term treatment of periodic depression with a mixture of sodium and lithium salts was proposed by the Danish internist Lange (1897). This was, however, never followed up by others and must therefore be regarded as a mere historical curiosity.

The real discovery and confirmation of the psychotropic properties of the lithium ion (Li^+) is credited to the Australian psychiatrists Cade (1949) and Noack and Trautner (1951). The Danish psychiatrist Strömgren noticed their papers, and their findings were reaffirmed by Schou et al. (1954).

The discovery that long-term treatment with Li^+ has a more or less complete repressive effect on the mood swings of patients suffering from episodes of manic-depressive illness of either the bipolar or the unipolar type was independently made by Hartigan (1963) and Baastrup (1964) and confirmed by cooperation between Baastrup and Schou (1967) and Baastrup et al. (1970). It is still a source of wonder that Li^+ should have no consistent effect on manifest endogenous depression.

Li^+ may furthermore have a favorable influence on morbid impulsive aggression and on emotional instability in children and adolescents. The ion may perhaps be useful in the treatment of granulocytopenia and thyrotoxic crisis.

The range of clinical uses of the lithium ion has been reviewed (Schou 1978).

THE URGENT NEED FOR SERUM-LEVEL MONITORING IN LITHIUM TREATMENT

Cade (1949) recognized the approach of intoxication. On the basis of his few patients he was able to describe almost ideally poisoning of moderate intensity and to urge in such cases immediate interruption of the treatment to avoid a fatal outcome. Furthermore, he noticed the crucial need for individualizing drug dosage. Noack and Trautner (1951) confirmed these facts:

"It is considered that the degree of lithium retention and the patient's tolerance to it determine the therapeutic effect. The lithium level necessary to terminate mania is probably always reached only by near-toxic dosage, but the two effects may not be closely related. Some patients do not suffer any toxic complications, while with others these symptoms may be grave enough to necessitate interruption of the medication before any effect on the mania is noticeable. These latter patients may, however, have their mania terminated if, after a few days, the treatment is recommenced at a lower, slowly increasing dosage. The question seems to be whether and how an efficient lithium level can be established."

Table 1 demonstrates that the dosages used today in long-term "prophylactic" treatment are of the same order of magnitude as those used for mania by Cade (1949) and Noack and Trautner (1951) and furthermore that the daily dosage differs within a wide range between patients.

It is essential to remember that the dosage necessary for one patient may be gravely toxic for another. It is furthermore remarkable that a therapeutic dosage showing no serious complications during extended periods of time may within a few days be changed into a toxic dosage by commonplace intercurrent ailments or conditions, which induce a moderate water or electrolyte depletion, such as fever, loss of appetite, slimming diet, hot weather, treatment with diuretics, and so on (Hansen and Amdisen 1978).

Fig. 1 shows our present opinion of the therapeutic range and its relation to toxicity when based on the standardized control measure "12h-stSli" (lithium concentration in the steady state in serum obtained twelve hours after the lase dose). The therapeutic range in fig. 1 represents the variation between individuals and concerns both the mood-swing repressing long-term treatment and the antimanic treatment according to table 1. This therapeutic range has not been titrated out through prospective studies; for several years it was based on clinical impression only (Schou et al. 1971); it was supported by deduction (Amdisen 1975a) from the less strictly standardized serum lithium concentration in the morning before the first

Table 1. Size of individualized daily dose of Li$^+$ in some major clinical trials as a psychotherapeutic drug.

Antimanic effect	
Cade (1949)	10–50 mmol
Roberts (1950)	Fatal poisoning after one week on about 40 mmol
Ashburner (1950)	About 50 mmol, in a few cases higher and in several lower
Noack and Trautner (1951)	20–50 mmol
Schou et al. (1954)	24–56 mmol
Relapse-repressive ("prophylactic") long-term treatment	
Baastrup et al. (1970)	12–80 mmol
Amdisen and Baastrup (1977)	8–54 mmol (cf. fig. 2)

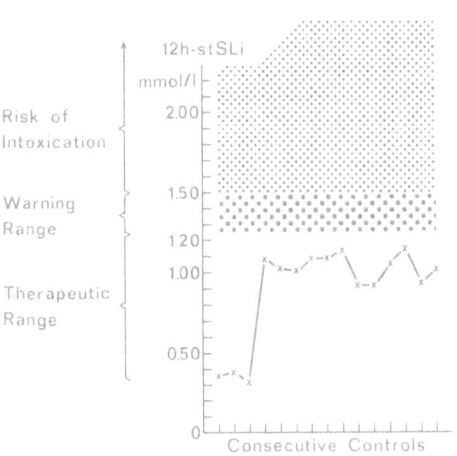

Figure 1. The significant ranges of 12h-stSLi. The curve of the figure demonstrates the check values of 12h-stSLi in a 42-year-old male during initiation and follow-up of lithium treatment. The first three controls were made on three consecutive weekdays after intake during the previous week of one Litarex ® tablet (6 mmol Li⁺) at 08.00 and 20.00. According to the values found the dosage was then increased to three Litarex ® tablets twice daily. The following four controls of 12h-stSLi correspond to once every week; the next five to once every month; and the rest to once every second or third month.

dose of the day (Amdisen 1967), and recently further by directly studying the 12h-stSli of 79 patients in successful long-term treatment (fig. 2).

Fig. 2 shows that the lowest and the highest placed responders differ by a factor of about three in respect to 12h-stSLi while the corresponding factor amounts to about 7 where the daily dose is concerned (Amdisen and Baastrup 1978). This is so because the dosage necessary to produce a certain level of 12h-stSLi depends on the renal lithium clearance as Li⁺ is almost solely eliminated from the human organism through the kidneys (Amdisen 1975a), and furthermore among normal subjects the renal lithium clearance varies by a factor of about four, 10–40 ml/min (Amdisen 1975a).

The serum concentration above which intoxication may occur (1.50 mmol/l) is also based only on clinical experience (Amdisen 1977; Hansen and Amdisen 1978). When 12h-stSLi is about 1.50 mmol/l the more sensitive patients demonstrate discrete, but for the "lithium-trained" clinician, unmistakable symptoms of intoxication, that is, some suggestion of the following symptoms: apathy or sluggishness, drowsiness, lethargy, sleepiness, difficulty in speaking, irregular tremor, myoclonic twitchings, muscular weakness, and ataxia (Amdisen and Schou 1978). The patient might at this lowest level of toxicity even "look ill, pinched, drawn, grey, and cold. Anorexia, nausea, and vomiting occur and occasionally diarrhoea" (Cade 1949). Gastrointestinal symptoms are, however, seldom encountered

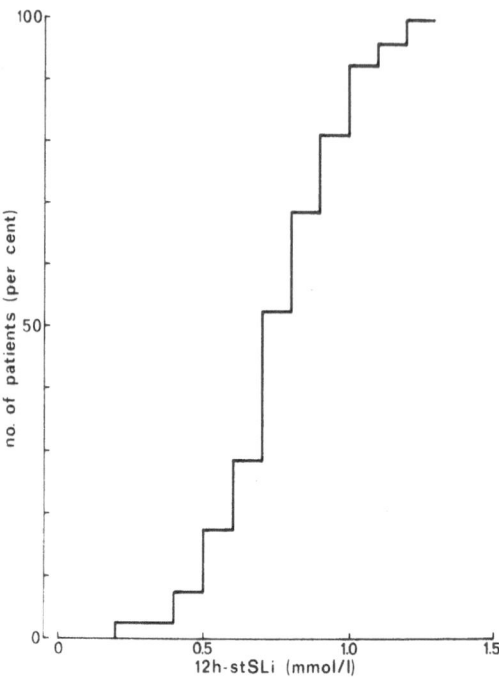

Figure 2. Cumulative frequency distribution of 79 patients in successful "prophylactic" lithium therapy according to their 12h-stSLi. All the patients were on several daily doses of conventional lithium carbonate or on controlled sustained-release tablets (either Litarex®, or Lithionit ® Durules ®). There were 63 females and 17 males aged 23 to 87 years. The daily dose ranged from 8 to 54 mmol Li$^+$ (Amdisen and Baastrup 1978).

in cases which have developed intoxication during long-term treatment, provided no recent increase of the dosage has taken place (Hansen and Amdisen 1978). In addition the renal toxicity of Li$^+$ itself, which impairs kidney function by a mechanism not yet understood, may appear at this only slightly elevated concentration level even in patients without any other symptoms of poisoning. If this has happened the patient has been caught in a vicious circle often leading to a grave intoxication, usually accompanied by more or less complete acute renal failure (Hansen and Amdisen 1978). This development may be interrupted if the patient has learned to recognize the syndrome of slight intoxication, immediately discontinues the treatment, and calls the doctor for control of 12h-stSLi.

It should be observed that Li$^+$, wherever present in the organism, must be considered as possessing its biological properties according to the actual concentration without any limitation, as it is neither protein-bound nor metabolized or detoxicated. Older animal data (Radomski et al. 1950; Evan and Ollerich 1972) and recent human data (Hestbech et al. 1977; Hansen et al. 1977; Hansen and Amdisen 1978) indicate that the distal part of the nephron may be exposed to damage as extreme Li^+ concentration of its luminal fluid is inevitable as the daily dose must be contained in the 24-hour urinary volume.

MONITORING METHODS IN LITHIUM TREATMENT

During the first 15–20 years of the history of Li^+ as a psychotropic drug the only means for adjustment of the individual dosage at start of treatment and during maintenance was a careful supervision of, on the one hand, symptoms of poisoning, and on the other hand, signs of too low a dosage. The former gave, as described by Noack and Trautner (1951), disturbing problems with some patients until it was generally appreciated that most patients adapted themselves to the slight toxic effects, so that after a temporary reduction, the dosage usually could be adequately increased within a few weeks. This unfortunately gave rise to the less frightening designation of "the initial side-effect" for this syndrome of slight intoxication, which was unfortunate, because later reappearance during treatment of this association of symptoms usually indicated a developing intoxication.

The task of finding an effective dosage for the individual patient solely by clinical observation of the disappearance of the disease was troublesome in treatment of mania, but became really difficult when the mood-swing repressing "prophylactic," long-term treatment was introduced in the mid-sixties, so there was an intensified search for supplementary valid guidance which would not require repeatedly pushing the patients into either slight poisoning or impending relapse.

Talbott (1950) claimed that lithium chloride might be safely used as a salt substitute provided the plasma or serum concentration never exceeded 1.00 mmol/l. Influenced by this Noack and Trautner (1951) and by them Schou et al. (1954) studied the correlation between serum concentration and pharmacodynamic effects. But their results were negative both in antimanic effect and adverse reactions. They came across patients with serum Li^+ concentration (SLi) close to 3.00 mmol/l with no discernible adverse reactions, and a severely intoxicated patient with SLi as low as 0.60 mmol/l. The majority of patients responding, however, usually presented SLi values lying between 0.50 and 2.00 mmol/l. Therefore that range of SLi was during the following years recommended as an admittedly rather weak supplement to clinical observation in monitoring of the treatment (Strömgren and Schou 1964).

It is readily understandable that the potential of SLi as a monitoring device was overlooked during this period; and with regard to procedure standardization the practical consequences of even the most simple pharmacokinetic properties of a drug were at that time not generally appreciated.

The reason for calling attention to these apparently obsolete matters is that in both scientific papers and textbooks one may still encounter SLi levels or SLi ranges without any specification of standardizing measures. This lack usually makes the information incomprehensible and may, as guidance, even be dangerous. From the following it appears that a situation with risk of intoxication may for example be present if a patient uses a regimen of one dose daily, with the blood sample for control of SLi being taken immediately before the dose intake (a "24h-stSLi") and adjustment of the dosage to give a control concentration within the upper part of the therapeutic range, 0.30–1.30 mmol/l. Peak concentrations may, in such cases reach a highly toxic level (see figs. 7 and 8).

The most important requirements of an SLi used for monitoring
There are two main requirements of an SLi used for monitoring. The first one is that intra-individually the control concentration should havè attained a reproducibility good enough to disclose the substantial concentration changes in emergency cases. A good reproducibility also enables a prophylactic unmasking of the more discrete increases of SLi which accompany both gradually decreasing kidney function and the slight kidney impairments produced by a negative fluid balance, and furthermore it enables the revealing of the greater instability found in cases of non-compliance. The second main demand is that the control value of different patients should be sufficiently comparable to permit dosage adjustment according to general experience of the therapeutic concentration range and that of risk of intoxication (fig. 1).

The necessity of avoiding the first ten hours in taking the control sample
Administered in a readily absorbable condition, as for example in a weak aqueous solution of the chloride, a dose of the lithium ion is directly transferred from the gastrointestinal tract via the bloodstream to a minor central part (15–20 percent) of its total apparent distribution volume. From the central compartment the dose is distributed to the peripheral compartment during the following eight to ten hours. Concomitantly a loss from the central compartment takes place through the kidneys with a velocity which is directly proportional to the actual plasma concentration of Li^+ (Amdisen 1975a).

The resulting SLi curve (fig. 3) shows a sudden rise to a high peak followed by a steep fall which after the point of final distribution, eight to ten hours later, continues as a less steep slope with a constant percentage decrease (semilogarithmically rectilinear). It should be noted that before the point of final distribution the SLi may at any time vary considerably as a result of rather small aberrations in the course of absorption. This is so because the deviations are reflected primarily to the smaller central com-

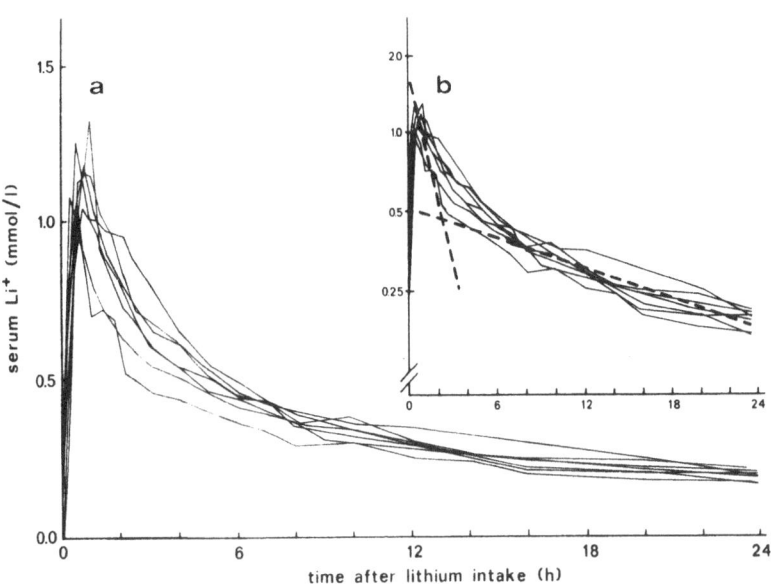

Figure 3. Twenty-four-hour course of the serum lithim concentration in seven healthy volunteers after the intake of 24 mmol Li$^+$ in a form of lithium chloride in 300 ml water: (a) conventional diagram: (b) semilogarithmic diagram (Amdisen 1975a).

partment. When the dose after the point of final distribution has been spread to the approximately seven times larger total apparent distribution volume these reflections from the course of absorption course are correspondingly attenuated.

This variation from time to time of the concentration course shortly after a dose intake is exaggerated by the environmental dependence of conventional tablets while a properly prepared controlled release preparation almost completely avoids this (fig. 4) and gives a higher time-to-time uniformity of the concentration course and thus the possibility of safer treatment control (Amdisen 1975b). For the patients who cannot cope with the *controlled sustained-release* tablets because of provoked diarrhoea it would be an advantage if a *controlled fast-release* tablet could be made available.

Fig. 5 exemplifies how an equal mean lithium concentration in serum may result in SLi values from a minimum of about 0.70 mmol/l to a maximum of more than 1.60 mmol/l if the blood sample is taken at incidental points during the day. But fig. 5 also suggests quite uniform concentration courses during the morning hours if the doses at 08.00 were omitted. The latter property can be exploited for establishing a control SLi.

Fig. 1 and fig. 6 show that blood samples taken in the morning before

A. AMDISEN

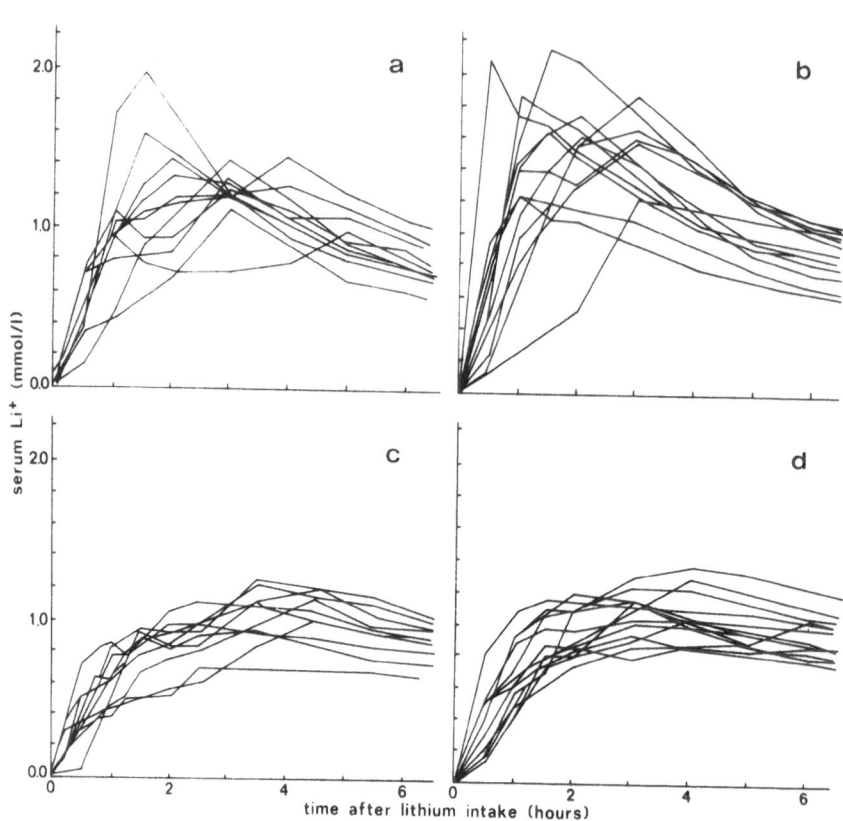

Figure 4. Course of serum lithium concentration during the absorption phase after the intake of a single dose of (a) and (b) conventional tablets, and (c) and (d) sustained-release tablets, under uniform experimental conditions, taking the tablets with light breakfast. For (a) and (c) about 0.70 mmol Li^+/kg body weight to 11 healthy volunteers; for (b) and (d) about 0.85 mmol Li^+/kg body weight to 12 volunteers; (a) conventional lithium carbonate tablets; (b) conventional lithium citrate tablets; (c) sustained-release tablets, Lithionit ® Durules ®; (d) sustained-release tablets, Litarex ® (Amdisen 1975a).

the first dose of the day and twelve hours after the evening dose present an intra-individual reproducibility sufficiently good for monitoring purposes.

THE DOSE REGIMEN

Fig. 7 demonstrates that dose schedules of more than one dose daily produce twelve-hour concentrations which are so much alike that their systematic differences are only of limited practical importance. The four times daily regimen has been omitted for the sake of clarity; it would have presented a 12h-stSLi of 0.96 mmol/l.

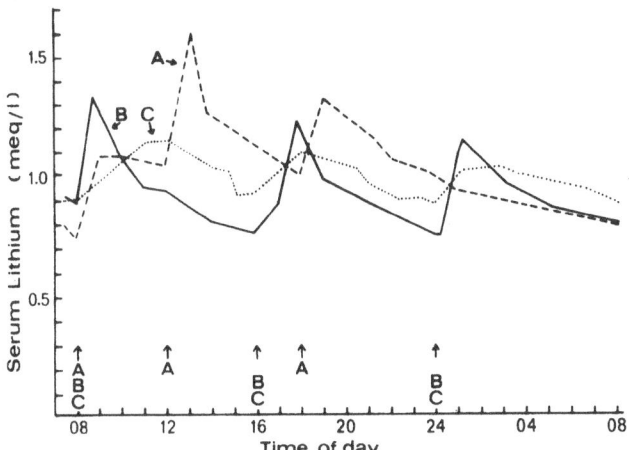

Figure 5. Three incidental serum lithium curves during the 24 hours of the day in the same 42-year-old male taking 12 mmol Li$^+$ thrice daily: A: conventional lithium carbonate tablets according to the conventional t.i.d. regimen; B: conventional lithium carbonate tablets every eight hour; and C: controlled sustained-release tablets Lithionit ® Durules ® every eighth hour.

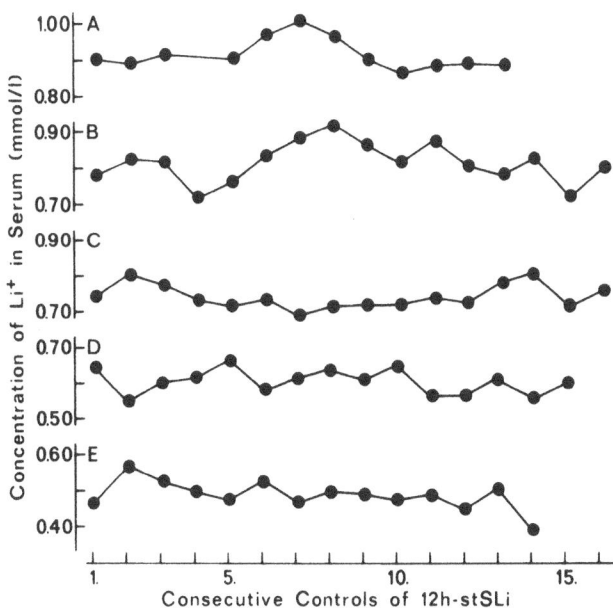

Figure 6. Twice-weekly check values of 12h-stSLi in five persons taking conventional lithium carbonate tablets (8.1 mmol Li$^+$ per tablet): A: two tablets at 08.00, one tablet at 14.00, and two tablets at 21.00; B: two tablets at 08.00, 14.00 and 21.00; C and D: one tablet at 08.00, 14.00 and 21.00: E: one tablet at 08.00 and 21.00.

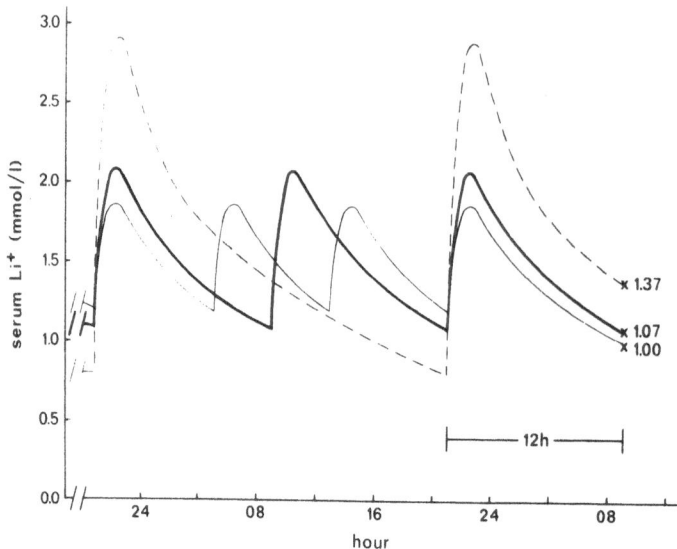

Figure 7. Computer-simulated concentration curves to illustrate the fundamental influence of the dosage schedule upon the 24-hour curve and upon the 12h-stSLi. The curves are constructed on the basis of the same 24-hour dose and $T_{1/2} = 13$ h, absorption rate corresponding to rapid absorption from conventional tablets – compare (a) and (b) of fig. 4 (Amdisen 1975a).

In addition Fig. 7 discloses the two main reasons for discarding the single dose regimen: first, its 12h-stSLi systematically deviates too much to permit use of the reference ranges for multiple dose schedules (fig. 1 and fig. 2) even when sustained-release tablets are concerned (fig. 8); secondly, this regimen produces a maximum concentration which is precariously high when considering the near-toxic mean level used in many cases.

Magnitude of the time interval between the last dose and taking of the control sample

The constant percentage decrease of SLi after the point of final distribution of the last dose is inversely proportional to the renal lithium clearance, which according to the admittedly rather sparse documentation may, in spite of a day to night variation (table 2), be regarded as intra-individually approximately constant. This fall rate, which can most simply be expressed as the half life, $T_{1/2}$, varies considerably however between subjects. In practice, as blood is sampled only during day this half-life is of interest in the present connection. Fig. 9 shows the distribution of subjects according to their $T_{1/2}$ and demonstrates a large inter-individual dispersion. The fundamental consequences of this for the SLi slopes during a day off lithium are illustrated in fig. 10. It appears that the longer the time interval is between the last dose

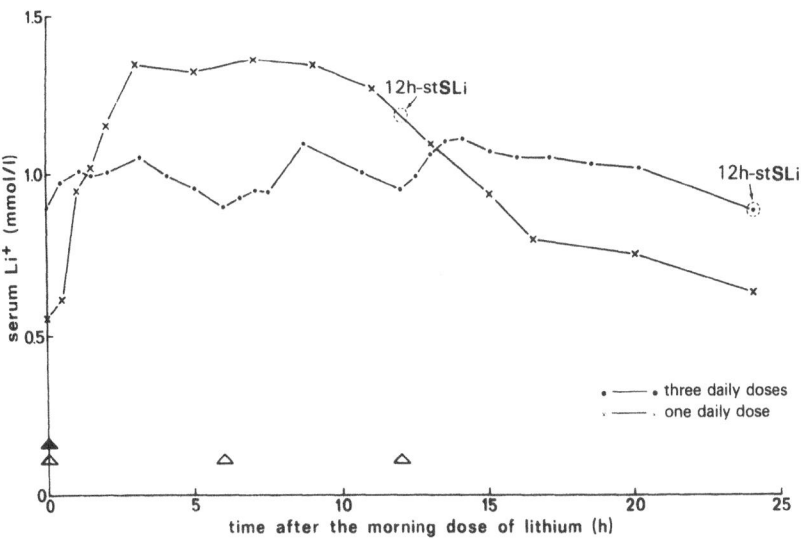

Figure 8; Twenty-four-hour serum lithium curves during steady state, on three daily doses and one daily dose, of controlled sustained-release tablets, Litarex ®: 12 mmol × 3 (△) and 36 mmol × 1 (▲) respectively, in a 51-year-old woman having $T_{1/2} = 14$h.

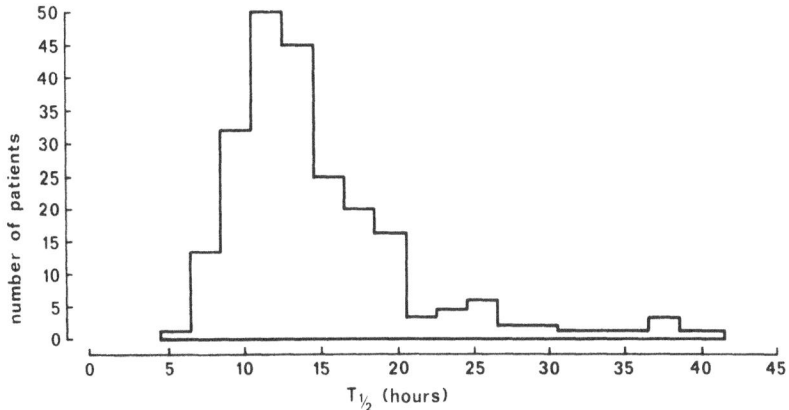

Figure 9. The frequency distribution of 177 patients and 49 healthy volunteers according to their $T_{1/2}$ (Amdisen 1975a).

and sampling the worse the SLi at a certain point of time can be compared between persons with equal mean SLi during the preceding time periods.

The twelve-hour interval, 12h-stSLi, has been chosen as the more appropriate compromise out of consideration for (1) the need of reasonable comparability between patients, which requires a shorter interval; (2)

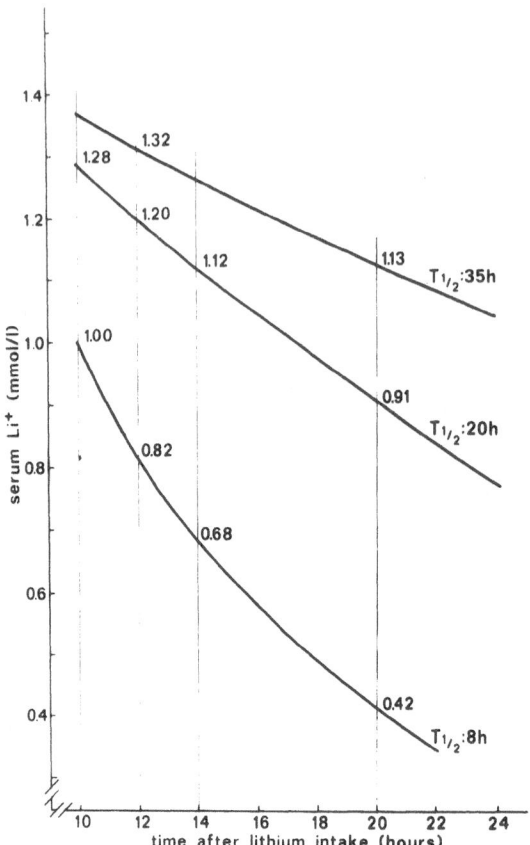

Figure 10. Computer-simulated serum lithium curves during a day without lithium, a "control day," for three "patients" showing characteristic $T_{1/2}$ values (cf. fig. 9). The curves were constructed presupposing the same mean serum level of lithium in steady state and presupposing the intake of two daily doses at accurate 12-hour intervals during the preceding days (Amdisen 1975a).

not too close dependence on the accuracy of the timing, which requires a less steep SLi slope and therefore a longer time interval; and (3) the rhythm of daily life.

It may be noticed that patients with steeper slopes (shorter $T_{1/2}$) should observe the twelve-hour timing more carefully (fig. 10). Such patients may be identified as subjects who need a relatively high dosage to achieve a certain level of 12h-stSLi.

Time of day for drawing of the control blood sample
There are at least three arguments for taking the control blood sample in the morning: (1) blood-taking in the afternoon or early evening twelve hours

after an early morning dose would not be especially convenient neither for the patient nor for the laboratory; (2) most patients have their dosage and concentration adjusted during stay in hospital by routine blood sampling in the morning; and (3) some patients show great differences in the SLi slope between night and day (table 2), and thus different 12h-stSLi values in the morning and evening.

Specification of the standardized control value

From the above it follows that the standardized control value, 12h-stSLi, is the concentration of Li^+ in serum or plasma of a blood sample drawn in the morning, before the first lithium dose of the day, 12 ± 0.5 hours after the evening dose from a patient complying completely with treatment in regard to dosage, dose regimen, and dose timing, taking the dosage in more than one dose per day, and who furthermore is in steady-state equilibrium of dosage and excretion.

The reproducibility of the 12h-stSLi demonstrated in fig. 1 and fig. 6 must be regarded as satisfactory for monitoring of the treatment. Attention should, however, be called to the fact that these results have been obtained in patients with good treatment compliance. The reliability of 12h-stSli as a protection against unintended changes of treatment conditions is crucially dependent on the patients complying with the doctor's instructions. The efforts required to establish perfect appreciation and cooperation from the patient cannot be overdone. Non-compliance in any of the respects mentioned above nullifies SLi as a monitoring device and may even make its use dangerous in cases of failing kidney function.

The actually existing variations in fig. 1 and fig. 6 furthermore disclose that a 12h-stSLi should not be regarded as an isolated observation, but

Table 2. Half-life $(T_{1/2})$ in hours for Li^+ during the day and during the night. All determinations done during the period 12 to 20 hours after the last dose of lithium (Amdisen 1975a).

Subject no.	Day	Night	Ratio: Night/day
1	13.5	15.5	1.15
2	11.0	13.0	1.18
3	10.5	14.0	1.33
4	14.0	19.0	1.36
5	13.5	21.0	1.56
6	11.5	18.0	1.57
7	12.0	20.0	1.67
8	8.0	15.0	1.88
9	11.0	22.0	2.00
10	10.5	24.0	2.29
11	13.5	33.5	2.48

evaluated in the light of previous values and repeated if any misgivings are present, several times if need be (Müller-Oerlinghausen 1977).

START OF LITHIUM TREATMENT

During initiation of lithium treatment or after a substantial change of dosage it is essential to investigate the mechanism of accumulation, that is, the increase of the concentration in spite of a constant daily dose until gradually the steady-state between intake and excretion has been achieved after a time period of approximately six times $T_{1/2}$ for a particular patient (fig. 11). Under conditions of equilibrium, steady-state conditions, there is a direct proportionality between daily dose and concentration level.

Start of long-term treatment
In the long-term situation there is ample time since the aim is to be achieved over months or years, a factor which should be used for the benefit of safety (Amdisen 1977). The patient should be instructed to take one lithium tablet exactly at, for example, 09.00 and 18.00 and to comply carefully. After a week 12h-stSLi should be checked on three consecutive weekdays. On the basis of these figures the dosage should be increased proportionally to give the desired 12h-stSLi.

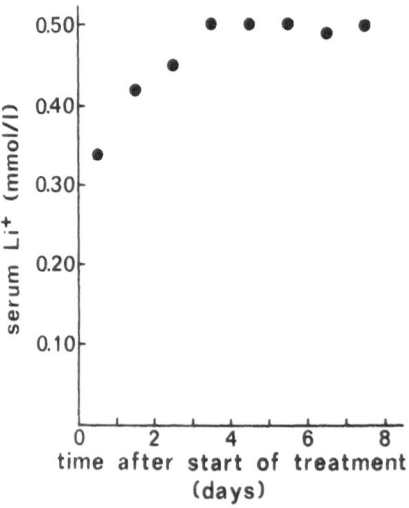

Figure 11. Serum lithium concentrations (12h-stSLi) during the establishment of steady state (period of accumulation), with administration of one daily dose of 24 mmol Li$^+$ in the form of a dilute solution of lithium chloride. $T_{1/2} = 15$ h (Amdisen 1975a).

With a patient commencing treatment, whose concentration requirements are unknown, the adjustment should aim at 0.80–1.00 mmol/l, because a majority of patients are severely disturbed by adverse reactions at the upper limit of the therapeutic range before the adaptation period has elapsed. But even after this only patients suffering from relapse should be pushed to the upper levels. The 12h-stSLi should then be checked once a week over the following months, montly for the next half year and from then about every second month (see example in fig. 1). This last is aimed at disclosing slowly developing kidney impairment, especially often encountered in the elderly.

The opportunity of frequent contact should be used to persuade the patient to appreciate the crucial importance of compliance for reliability of of the 12h-stSLi and thus for the safety of this near-toxic treatment. Furthermore, to avoid severe intoxication in case of intercurrent ailment, the contacts should be exploited to train the patient to recognize with certainty the associated symptoms of slight intoxication.

Start of acute treatment

In cases of mania the steady-state level of 12h-stSLi may be reached rapidly by using booster dosages for the first three or four days: for example a daily dose of 40–50 mmol Li^+. The 12h-stSLi should be checked daily, evaluated with consideration of the steady-state mechanism, and the dosage changed accordingly. The potential benefit of this procedure seems evident but has not been confirmed by systematic investigation. After this initial phase the 12h-stSLi and the patient should be handled as in long-term treatment.

USE OF SERUM LITHIUM CONCENTRATION DATA IN CASE OF
LITHIUM POISONING

A common feature of the course of lithium intoxication is a dissociation of time between the toxic SLi levels and their symptoms. The resulting lag period may even amount to several days (Amdisen et al. 1974; Ashong et al. 1975; Hansen and Amdisen 1978). On admission to hospital the patient may present intoxication symptoms of moderate intensity only and have an apparently corresponding and not too alarming SLi. But in spite of a continuous, although usually rather slow, decrease of SLi the patient's condition may during the following hours or days worsen and the outcome may be fatal.

In most such cases it may be that the last dose of lithium was taken many hours or a few days ago, and the fall of SLi may disclose that the lithium concentration has been at real toxic levels prior to the admittance to hospital. Therefore, at the slightest suspicion of lithium poisoning, the procedure should be as follows:

1. A blood sample should be taken immediately and the analysis carried out urgently.

2. Information concerning the time of last lithium intake and the size of the dose should be intensively sought.

3. The serum lithium estimation should be repeated every three hours and the figures plotted on a semilog diagram.

If interpretation of this information reveals that (1) SLi has not during the time after the point of final distribution of the last dose been above 2.50 mmol/l and (2) the consecutive SLi values drawn every third hour indicate achievement of an SLi lower than 1.00 mmol/l within 30 hours after commencement of the emergency, the patient may be treated conservatively with especial concern for fluid balance – many lithium patients undoubtedly are prone to a negative water balance because of polyuria, or even impaired concentrating ability, induced by the long-term lithium treatment (Hansen et al. 1977; Hansen and Amdisen 1978).

If the demands mentioned cannot be satisfied the patient should be treated urgently with hemodialysis, which should be repeated until the SLi has been brought below 1.00 mmol/l, when estimated at the approximate point of final redistribution, six hours after finishing the hemodialysis – see

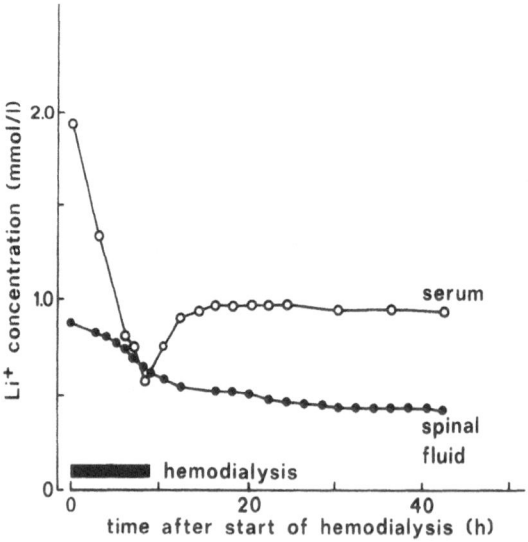

Figure 12. Li$^+$ concentrations in serum and spinal fluid during and after hemodialysis of a severely intoxicated 65-year-old male.

figs. 12 and 13) (Hansen and Amdisen 1978). Peritoneal dialysis should be used only if hemodialysis facilities are not available.

CONCLUSIONS

The dosage requirements of the lithium ion (Li^+), which is the active agent of the lithium salts used in therapy, should always be regarded as near-toxic. The dose varies considerably inter-individually, so much that the therapeutic dosage of one patient may be highly toxic for another. Furthermore commonplace ailments may change the dosage used from therapeutic to toxic.

Until about fifteen years ago the Li^+ concentration in serum, or plasma, had in monitoring of the treatment to be considered as a rather unreliable supplement to clinical awareness of on the one hand symptoms of impending intoxication and on the other hand signs of inadequate dosage.

Through standardization of the conditions under which the blood sample is taken the serum lithium concentration can be converted to become the main monitoring device in lithium treatment. The most important variables to be controlled are the time interval between last dose and blood taking, the dose schedule, and the time of day.

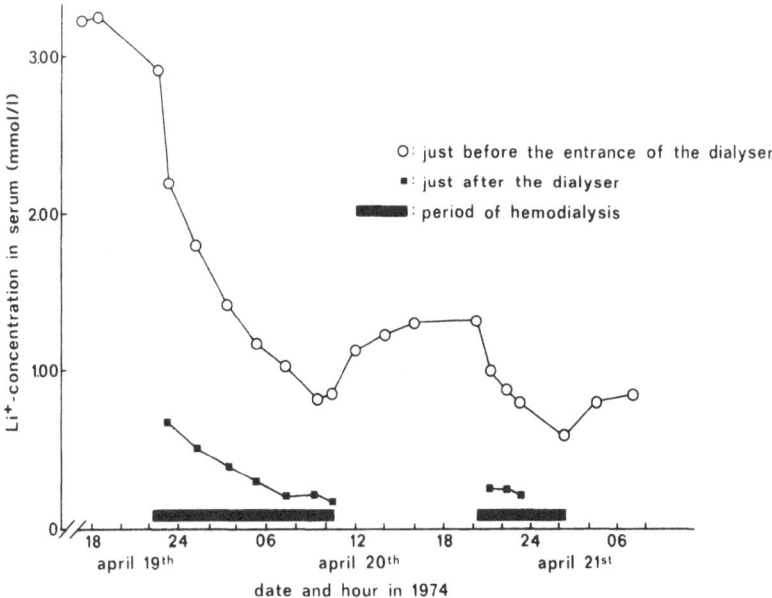

Figure 13. Li^+ concentration in serum before, during, and after hemodialysis of a severely intoxicated 66-year-old male.

The therapeutic concentrations of lithium in the steady state in serum obtained 12h after the last dose (12h-stSLi), are in the range of 0.30–1.30 mmol/l. The vicious circle of intoxication might start at 1.50 mmol/l.

The lithium ion concentration is indispensable both for the diagnosis and the treatment regime of lithium intoxication.

Despite of use of 12h-stSLi as a means of monitoring, the patient should be trained in recognizing the symptom association of poisoning of moderate intensity: speech difficulty, irregular tremor, myoclonic twitchings, muscular weakness, and ataxia.

REFERENCES

Amdisen, A., Serum lithium determinations for clinical use. *Scand. J. Clin. Lab. Invest.* 20, 104–108 (1967).

Amdisen, A., Monitoring of lithium treatment through determination of the serum lithium concentration. *Dan. Med. Bull.* 22, 277–291 (1975a).

Amdisen, A., Sustained-release preparations of lithium. In: *Lithium Research and Therapy.* Ed., Johnson, F.N., London, 1975b, pp. 197–210.

Amdisen, A., Serum level monitoring and clinical pharmacokinetics of lithium. *Clinical Pharmacokinetics* 2, 73–92 (1977).

Amdisen, A., Gottfries, C.G., Jacobsson, L. and Winblad, B., Grave lithium intoxication with fatal outcome. *Acta Psychiat. Scand. (Suppl).* 255, 25–33 (1974).

Amdisen, A. and Schou, M., Lithium. In: *Side Effects of Drugs Annual* 2. Ed., Dukes, M.N.G., Amsterdam, 1978, pp. 17–29.

Ashburner, J.V., A case of chronic mania treated with lithium citrate and terminating fatally – correspondence to Roberts. *Med. J. Aust.* 37, 386 (1950).

Ashong, M.R., Fernandez, P.G. and McLeod, P.J., Fatal self-poisoning with lithium carbonate. *Canad. Med. Ass. J.* 112, 868–870 (1975).

Baastrup, P.C., The use of lithium in manic-depressive psychosis. *Comprehens. Psychiat.* 5, 396-408 (1964).

Baastrup, P.C., Poulsen, J.C., Schou, M., Thomsen, K. and Amdisen, A., Prophylactic lithium: double-blind discontinuation in manic-depressive and recurrent-depressive disorders. *Lancet* 2, 326–330 (1970).

Baastrup, P.C. and Schou, M., Lithium as a prophylactic agent: its effect against recurrent depression and manic-depressive psychosis. *Arch. Gen. Psychiat.* 16, 162–172 (1967).

Cade, J.F.J., Lithium salts in the treatment of psychotic excitement. *Med. J. Aust.* 36, 349–352 (1949).

Evan, A.P. and Ollerich, D.A., The effect of lithium carbonate on the structure of the rat kidney. *Amer. J. Anat.* 134, 97–106 (1972).

Hansen, H.E. and Amdisen, A., Lithium intoxication (report of 23 cases and review of 100 cases from the literature). *Quart. J. Med.* 47, 123–144 (1978).

Hansen, H.E., Hestbech, J., Olsen, S. and Amdisen, A., Renal function and renal pathology in patients with lithium-induced impairment of renal concentrating ability. *Proc. Eur. Dial. Transp. Ass.* 14, 518–527 (1977).

Hartigan, G.P., The use of lithium salts in affective disorders. *Brit. J. Psychiat.* 109, 810–814 (1963).

Hestbech, J., Hansen, H.E., Amdisen, A. and Olsen, S., Chronic renal lesions following long-term treatment with lithium. *Kidney Int.* 12, 205–213 (1977).

Lange, C., Bidrag til Urinsyrediatesens Klinik. *Hospitalstidende* 5, 21–38 (1897).

Müller-Oerlinghausen, B., 10 Jahre Lithium-Katamnese. *Nervenarzt* 48, 483–493 (1977).

Noack, C.H. and Trautner, E.M., The lithium treatment of maniacal psychosis. *Med. J. Aust.* 38, 219–222 (1951).

Radomski, J.L., Fuyat, H.N., Nelson, A.A. and Smith, P.K., The toxic effects, excretion, and distribution of lithium chloride. *J. Pharmacol. Exp. Ther.* 100, 429–444 (1950).

Roberts, E.L., A case of chronic mania treated with lithium citrate and terminating fatally. *Med. J. Aust.* 37, 261 (1950).

Schou, M., The range of clinical uses of lithium. In: *Lithium in Medical Practice*. Ed., Johnson, F.N. and Johnson, S., Lancaster, 1978, pp. 21–39.

Schou, M., Amdisen, A. and Baastrup, P.C., The practical management of lithium treatment. *Brit. J. Hosp. Med.* 6, 53–60 (1971).

Schou, M., Juel-Nielsen, N., Strömgren, E. and Voldby, H., The treatment of manic psychoses by the administration of lithium salts. *J. Neurol. Neurosurg. Psychiat.* 17, 250–260 (1954).

Strömgren, E. and Schou, M., Lithium treatment of manic states. *Postgrad. Med.* 35, 83–86 (1964).

Talbott, J.H., Use of lithium salts as a substitute for sodium chloride. *Arch. Intern. Med.* 85, 1–10 (1950).

7. TRICYCLIC ANTIDEPRESSANTS

P. KRAGH-SØRENSEN

Tricyclic antidepressants (TAs) came into clinical use nearly twenty years ago. Their clinical efficacy has been established beyond doubt but their therapeutic effect varies considerably from patient to patient and from study to study (Bennett 1967). Several investigators have performed controlled trials to compare different TAs, but no clear-cut nor consistent clinical differences between the various compounds have emerged. However, some characteristics associated with therapy are recognized:

1. The therapeutic effect is usually most clearly drug-related in patients suffering from so-called endogenous depression;

2. The onset of therapeutic effect is normally delayed two to six weeks;

3. Treatment with these drugs gives a recovery rate of about sixty percent (Morris and Beck 1974);

4. Overdoses of TA often produce severe toxic symptoms, especially of a cardiovascular nature.

Until the beginning of the 1970s, the individual variability in therapeutic effect was studied mainly as a function of differences in clinical symptomatology (Hollister 1972, 1973), and very little attention was paid to the problem of dosage. Some investigators claim that a positive effect is often obtained only with very high doses, for example 200–300 mg daily or more (Pöldinger 1964).

Most psychiatrists would probably agree that the dosage of TAs should be individually assessed for each patient. In clinical practice this adjustment can be made on the basis of therapeutic effect or the demonstration of side-effects, but these parameters are inconclusive because, firstly, the onset of clinical effect is normally delayed – a factor which is time-consuming, and secondly because of difficulties in distinguishing between the side effects and depressive symptoms.

These problems are also well-known in other fields of medicine, such as in the treatment of epilepsy with antiepileptic drugs and treatment of cardiovascular disorders with digoxin. The determination of drug concentration in plasma has often proved a valuable aid in these therapeutic situations and the demonstration of pronounced inter-individual variation in the steady-state plasma level of TAs suggests that the variability in therapeutic effect may be related to the drug concentration in plasma (see fig. 1).

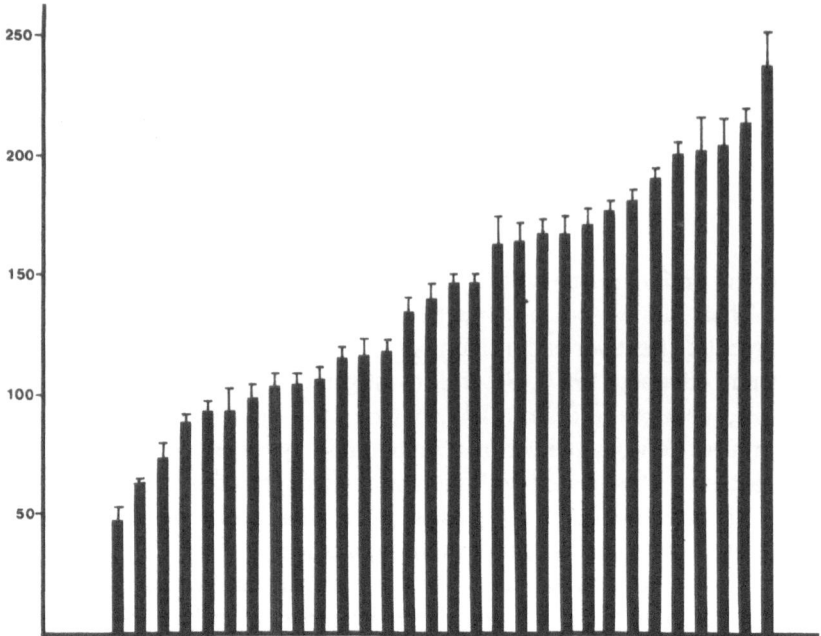

Figure 1. Steady-state plasma concentrations of nortriptyline (μg/l). **Mean and standard error** of six determinations from the second to the fourth weeks in thirty patients with endogenous depression treated with 50 mg nortriptyline t.i.d (**Kragh-Sørensen et al. 1973**).

PHARMACOKINETIC PROPERTIES

Today sufficiently sensitive analytical methods are available for the determination of all known TA drugs in plasma (Gram 1977a). and the pharmacokinetic properties of these drugs have been thoroughly studied since the beginning of the 1970s, both clinically and experimentally (Alexanderson 1972; von Bahr 1972; Gram 1974).

The following relevant clinical data can be extracted from these studies:

1. TAs have a high degree of *tissue binding*, with an apparent volume of distribution in the range of 10 to 20 l/kg.

2. There is efficient elimination by hepatic metabolism with a *systemic clearance* of 300–1200 ml/min. The combination of the large volume of distribution and the high systemic clearance results in plasma half-life ($T_{1/2}$ of intermediate length, but there are marked differences between individuals and between drugs e.g. for imipramine $T_{1/2} = 6$–20 h, for nortriptyline $T_{1/2} = 15$–90 h). The inter-individual variation in plasma steady-state concentration is mainly due to the inter-individual variation in clearance.

3. Another factor which influences these variations is *protein binding*, which ranges from 75–97 percent with both inter-individual and inter-drug differences (Glassman et al. 1973; Kragh-Sørensen, Hansen, et al. 1976).

4. It is known that in any given individual, the plasma concentration of a particular TA is a personal characteristic, and remains stable and reproducible unless other drugs are given simultaneously. This is to be expected, as the steady-state concentration level is to a great extent under *genetic control* (Alexanderson 1973).

CLINICAL EFFECTS AND PLASMA LEVELS

Pharmacokinetic information is of great importance in clinical pharmacological studies where the correlation between plasma concentration and clinical effects of a drug is sought.

During the past six to eight years several groups have correlated pharmacokinetic properties, in particular steady-state plasma levels, with clinical effects (see Gram 1977a). These efforts have centred on the *antidepressive* effect, whereas *side effects* and *toxicity* have been given less attention. To date more than fifteen studies have been carried out in various parts of the world and more than 600 patients have been examined in an attempt to determine the correlation between plasma concentrations of different TAs and therapeutic effect. All known TA drugs have been investigated but in spite of all this work it must be concluded that for most of these drugs, plasma level monitoring for TA therapy remains a field open to research. Knowledge of two drugs, however, namely nortriptyline and imipramine, is such that today plasma level monitoring of the compound can be recommended.

METHODOLOGY: CLINICAL PHARMACOLOGICAL PROBLEMS

The subject of this paper mainly concerns the general reluctance to accept plasma measurements of TAs as part of clinical psychiatry. As mentioned above only sixty percent of the patients treated with TAs are said to respond satisfactorily to treatment. From a kinetic point of view it would be natural to conclude that the reason approximately one third of the patients in earlier investigations did not respond to the treatment prescribed was that the plasma concentration was inadequate and that this resulted from incorrect dosage. However, such a simple conclusion is not acceptable. It is necessary to point out that the intense clinical kinetic research work carried out in latter years has also made it possible to put forward a number of minimum requirements which are more or less satisfied in some recent investigations.

Analytical methods
It is necessary to emphasize the importance of efficient analytical and technical facilities. The steady-state plasma levels of TAs given in conventional dosages are relatively low, namely from 20–900 μg/l. This is an indication of how difficult the development of assay techniques for clinical use would be. None of the existing *chromatographic techniques* is immediately available in a routine laboratory and maintenance requires some analytical expertise. *Radioimmunoassay techniques* have not yet been developed for routine use in daily clinical work. Another factor to be considered is the possible inconsistency of the different techniques used in the various studies, as consistency has been achieved in only a few cases. Where a parent substance and active metabolite(s) are present, it is also important that specific methods of measurement are available for both/all substances.

Pharmacokinetics
The next requirement is complete knowledge of the pharmacokinetics of the particular TA. Application of this knowledge should be based on the theory that there is a constant relation between receptor site and plasma concentration in a particular individual. The condition is probably fulfilled with regard to that portion of the drug which is not protein-bound, but for practical reasons TAs have been measured as the total drug in plasma. Some studies have a two- to threefold shown inter-individual variation in the free fraction for desipramine and nortriptyline (Alexanderson and Borgå 1972; Burrows et al. 1974; Kragh-Sørensen, Hansen et al. 1976; Sjöqvist et al. 1969) and for imipramine a factor of 4.5 has been reported (Glassman et al 1973). The practical implication of this variability in its relation to therapeutic effect has not yet been studied, but it can perhaps explain why the results obtained for some TAs may be described as confusing.

Dosage
Another clinical pharmacological problem concerns dosage schedules. This problem is related to length of time between last drug intake and blood sampling, definition of steady state, and knowledge of the actual plasma half-life of the parent drug and metabolites. Generally it can be concluded that the plasma half-life of these drugs is relatively long (6–90 h). This again indicates that a dosage schedule of once to twice daily can be recommended. With regard to blood sampling after the last drug intake, we do not know anything regarding the time needed to reach equilibrium between receptor and plasma. Concentration curves following oral and

intravenous administration of TAs indicate that absorption and distribution may take as long as 3–8 h (Gram et al. 1976; Kragh-Sørensen, Borgå et al. 1977). It seems advisable, therefore, to sample blood ten to fifteen hours after last drug intake.

Depending on the drug, patient characteristics and environmental factors, steady-state plasma levels can be achieved within one to four weeks (Alexanderson 1972; Aasberg, Cronholm et al. 1971, Gram et al. 1977). The plasma concentration remains fairly stable over a period of months or years (Kragh-Sørensen et al. 1974 and Kragh-Sørensen, Hansen et al. 1976) and the fluctuations within dosage intervals are small – 10–20 percent (see figs. 2 and 3).

It is known that concurrent administration of other psychotherapeutic drugs may interfere with the kinetics of TAs. Barbiturates cause a drop in plasma levels (Sjöqvist 1971), and various phenothiazines as well as haloperidol inhibit the metabolism of TAs and may therby cause elevation of plasma levels of the drug see fig. 4 (Gram et al. 1977b; Kragh-Sørensen, Borgå et al. 1977).

Patient selection

The greatest methodological errors occur in the patient selection procedure, errors that lead to the inconsistencies found in results available in the literature. In psychiatry there is no clear-cut worldwide diagnostic classification system. In this type of research, it has therefore been necessary to

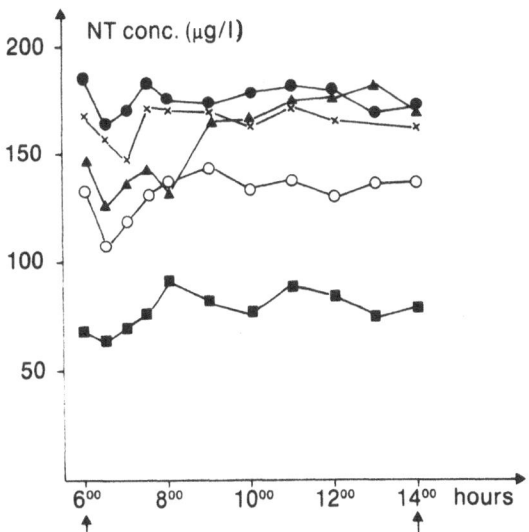

Figure 2.   Plasma levels of nortriptyline (NT) during an eight-hour dose interval (06.00–14.00) in five female patients on continuous treatment (Kragh-Sørensen et al. 1974).

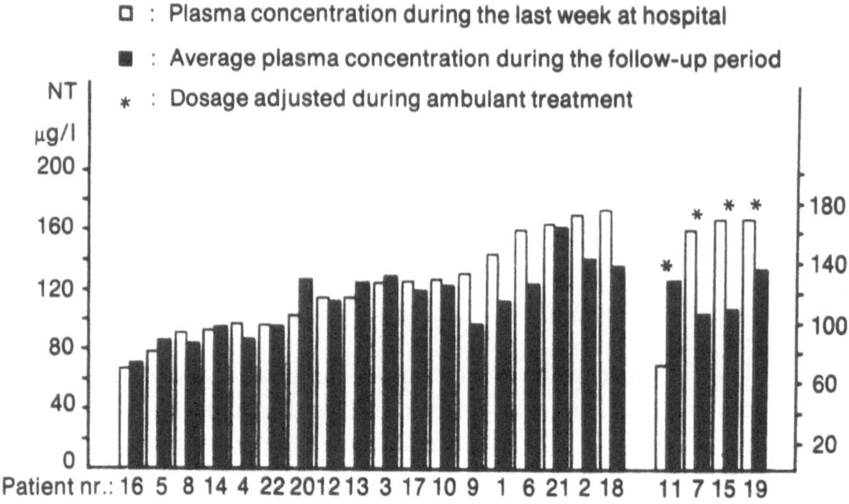

□ : Plasma concentration during the last week at hospital

■ : Average plasma concentration during the follow-up period

* : Dosage adjusted during ambulant treatment

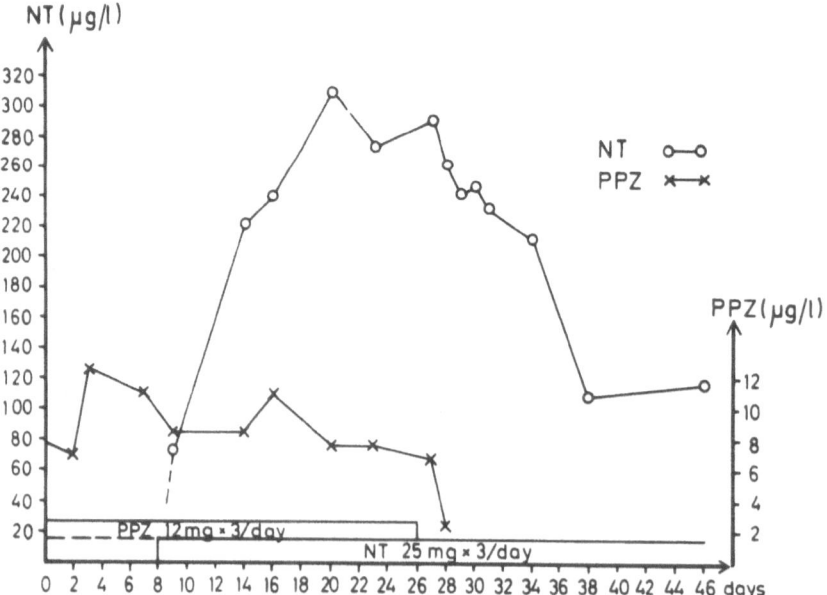

Figure 3. Plasma levels of 22 patients with endogenous depression treated with nortriptyline during the last week in hospital and the follow-up period (six months) respectively (Kragh-Sørensen et al. 1974).

Figure 4. Effect of concomitant perphenazine (PPZ) administration on nortriptyline (NT) plasma levels.

use so-called qualitative, or diagnostic, rating scales (Gurney et al. 1972). In this way results obtained are reliable within the clinic, the country, and across national borders.

While the diagnostic or qualitative rating scales are not generally accepted, the use of quantitative rating scales is. In the absence of biochemical parameters with a proven relationship to degree of depression, a scientific study of antidepressive effect has to be based on quantitative rating scales (Hamilton 1972; Cronholm and Ottosson 1960; Aasberg et al. 1973). The use of total scores on these rating scales has proved to be applicable and valid and is considered a better measurement of antidepressant treatment than the so-called global or clinical assessment (Bech et al. 1975).

Other factors
The placebo period, the duration of treatment, and the statistical analysis of the results, are other factors which are of great importance and which vary from one investigation to another (Kragh-Sørensen, Hansen et al. 1976).

PRACTICAL CLINICAL OBSERVATIONS

With these considerable methodological problems in mind it is almost impossible to correlate published studies because of their varying design. The inconsistency in results should, therefore, be considered in the light of the methodological problems mentioned.

Therapeutic plasma range
It can be said today that a therapeutic plasma range has been worked out for nortiptyline and imipramine only. The plasma range for nortriptyline is between 50 and 150 $\mu g/l$, and this means that plasma levels which are too low or too high, result in poor therapeutic effect (Kragh-Sørensen et al. 1973; Kragh-Sørensen et al. 1976; Ziegler et al. 1976; Montgomery et al. 1978).

It studies on imipramine a lower limit of therapeutic effect was found for the parent drug ($45\mu g/l$) with 75 $\mu g/l$ for its metabolite desipramine (Gram et al. 1976; Reisby et al. 1977). Poor response was seen more frequently in patients with low levels and no indication that high plasma levels and poor therapeutic effect are associated was found.

Several investigators have tried to correlate other TA plasma concentrations with therapeutic effect but results are inconclusive because of the investigational designs used. This is particularly a problem in studies attempting to bring to light a correlation between clinical effects and amitriptyline plasma concentrations (Braithwaite et al. 1972; Montgomery and Braithwaite 1975; Ziegler, Clayton et al. 1976; Kupfer et al. 1977; Coppen et al. 1978).

Cost benefit
Fulfilment of the minimal requirements, in clinical kinetic investigations of TAs, has resulted in greater certainty when recommending the use of measurements of plasma concentration of the particular drug in daily clinical practice. However, for many reasons, among which those already mentioned, plasma measurement is only carried out in very few institutions It is, of course, not surprising that many clinicians are sceptical of available research studies and have difficulty in acknowledging the relevance of introducing drug assays as a necessary requirement in clinical practice. To a certain extent this scepticism is well founded. It cannot be claimed that, because technical analysis methods exist and therapeutic plasma concentration areas have been found for a particular drug, investment in a routine analysis programme should necessarily follow. Such a decision probably depends on a cost-benefit analysis in which the patient's, the doctor's and society's benefits are compared with the cost, risks and disadvantages involved for these groups. Apart from this, evaluation of the practical advantages and consequences of these measurements is desirable, but it is hardly possible to perform this product control in all its phases. It is troublesome, time-consuming, and difficult to supervise. However, an attempt should be made to evaluate the practical advantages and disadvantages and in particular the consequences for the patient and thereby indirectly for the doctor. Investigations explicitly concerned with these practical problems have been carried out only in the case of nortriptyline (Braithwaite et al. 1972; Sørensen et al. 1978). They are especially concerned with diagnostics, dosage, and plasma monitoring in the clinical situation.

CONTROL OF THERAPY

With regard to plasma monitoring attention has been specifically directed to the question in which clinical situations and with which patients monitoring should be undertaken.

Risk groups
In the treatment of elderly patients many clinicians prefer ECT therapy because of the cardiotoxicity of TAs. But this dangerous side effect only occurs in patients with high plasma levels, and in the case of nortriptyline, over a limit of 200 μg/l. The therapeutic effects in elderly patients (in the age group of about 65 years) are as satisfactory as in younger persons (Søren-

sen et al. 1978) and treatment can be carried out without cardiovascular problems when nortriptyline plasma concentrations are in the area of 100 μg/1. Treatment can also be given to patients with cardiac diseases, provided plasma concentrations are carefully controlled during hospitalization.

Therapeutic problems
The therapeutic effect achieved after about two weeks treatment is a reliable predictor (Gram et al. 1976; Moody et al. 1977). Plasma monitoring in the third week of treatment is, therefore, indicated in many cases, and especially in those where the initial effect is absent (Sørensen et al. 1978).

With regard to side effects, many patients discontinue their medication because of several constant, but harmless, side effects. This often occurs in the early stage of treatment, when difficulty in distinguishing between side effects and depressive symptoms is greatest.

Maintenance therapy
It should be remembered when dealing with control of therapy that antidepressive treatment with a TA is symptomatic and not causal. From early literature it is known that a depressive phase can last an average of three to six months. Maintenance therapy should therefore continue for at least six months. From a pharmacokinetic point of view and supported by the conclusions reached in recent studies (Kragh-Sørensen et al. 1974; Kragh-Sørensen, Hvidberg et al. 1976), the problem can be summarized as follows:

1. Nortriptyline does not accumulate in the body during long-term treatment, so

a. plasma levels inside the therapeutic range (50–150 μg/l) can be kept constant for years on the same dose;

b. a reduced dose during long-term treatment is not justified from a clinical-pharmacological point of view.

2. Prevention of new episodes in unipolar manic-depressive disease is associated with therapeutic control and maintenance of the plasma concentration inside the therapeutic range.

As a result of these clinical kinetic investigations it is possible to produce data applicable in the clinical treatment of patients with so-called endogenous depression.

The starting point of these investigations was to show the great individual differences in the metabolism of TAs. Today the importance of these kinetic data in clinical effect is very clear, but the investigations have also shown that the study of kinetics alone has only brought us a little closer the actual target, namely to ensure the patient with an endogenous depression a speedy, satisfactory, and 100-percent active treatment.

CONCLUSION

With the exception of nortriptyline, more extensive studies on all TAs are necessary. These studies should cover larger patient populations with varying diagnostic categories and age and risk groups. Studies on the importance of protein binding in plasma in therapeutic effect should be given high priority, and there is a pressing need for development of feasible techniques for therapy control, both during hospitalization and in out-patient treatment.

On the basis of results built explicitly on practical treatment problems in daily clinical work, it seems justifiable to recommend, regardless of dosage policy, control of the plasma level at least once during the course of a hospital treatment with nortriptyline. Preferably it should be done in the second week, so as to maintain the plasma level within the optimal range of 50–150 μg/l if possible, aiming at a level of about 100 μg/l. The assay used for plasma determinations of nortriptyline must be dependable and carried out as a routine analysis in the laboratory, and the medical staff must be trained to interpret the consequences of the plasma concentration results. If this is to be made possible, a departmental strategy for such monitoring must be developed as part of the routine treatment of patients with endogenous depression.

If this procedure were followed, about 85–90 percent of those patients treated with nortriptyline within the therapeutic plasma concentration range would recover during a treatment period of four to six weeks.

For imipramine too, a relationship between plasma level and therapeutic effect has been demonstrated. The recommended plasma range for this is $> 45\,\mu$g/l, and $> 75\,\mu$g/l for its active metabolite desipramine.

Diagnostic problems in psychiatry are still a great hindrance to the achievement of 100-percent effective treatment and the need for objective biological parameters, possibly based on the so-called monoamine theory (Carlsson 1976) is evident.

REFERENCES

Aasberg, M., Cronholm, B., Sjöqvist, F. and Tuck, D., Relationship between plasma level and therapeutic effect of nortriptyline *British Medical Journal* 3, 331–334 (1971).

Aasberg, M., Evans, D.A.P., Sjöqvist, F. Genetic control of nortriptyline kinetics in man: a study of relatives of propositi with high plasma concentrations. *Journal of Medical Genetics* 8, 129–135 (1971).

Aasberg, M., Kragh-Sørensen, P., Mindham, R.H.S., Tuck, D., International reliability and communicability of a rating scale for depression. *Psychological Medicine* 3, 458–465 (1973).

Alexanderson, B., Pharmacokinetics of desmethylimipramine and nortriptyline in man after single and multiple oral doses. *European Journal of Clinical Pharmacology* 5, 1–10 (1972).

Alexanderson, B., Prediction of steady-state plasma levels of nortriptyline from single oral dose kinetics: a study in twins. *European Journal of Clinical Pharmacology* 6, 44–53 (1973).

Alexanderson, B. and Borgå, O., Interindividual differences in plasma protein binding of nortriptyline in man: a twin study. *European Journal of Clinical Pharmacology* 4, 196–200 (1972).

Bahr, C. von., Metabolism of tricyclic antidepressants: pharmacokinetic and molecular aspects." Thesis, Stockholm, 1972.

Bech, P., Gram, L.F., Dein, E., Jacobsen, O., Vitger, J. and Bolwig, T.G. Quantitative rating of depressive states. *Acta Psychiatrica Scandinavica* 51, 161–170 (1975).

Bennett, J.F., Is there a superior antidepressant? In: *Antidepressant Drugs*. Ed., Garattini and Dukes (Excerpta Medica Amsterdam, 1967), pp. 375–393.

Braithwaite, R.A., Goulding, R., Theano, G., Nailey, J. and Coppen, A., Plasma concentration of amitriptyline and clinical response. *Lancet* 1, 1297–1300 (1972).

Burrows, G.D., Scoggins, B.A. and Davies, B., Plasma nortriptyline and clinical response. In: *Classification and Prediction of Outcome of Depression: Symposium*. Ed., Angst, Stuttgart, 1974, pp. 178–179.

Carlsson, A. The contribution of drug research to investigating the nature of endogenous depression. *Pharmakopsychiatrie* 9, 2–10 (1976).

Coppen, A., Montgomery, S., Ghose, K., Rama Rao, V.A., Bailey, J., Christiansen, J., Mikkelsen P.L., van Praag, H.M., van de Poel, F., Minsker, E.J., Kozulja, V.G., Matussek, N., Kungkunz, G. and Jørgensen, A., Amitriptyline plasma-concentration and clinical effect: a World Health Organization collaborative study. *Lancet*, January 14, 1978.

Cronholm, B. and Ottoson, J.O., Experimental studies of the therapeutic action of electroconvulsive therapy in endogenous depression. *Acta Scandinavica* 35, suppl. 145, 69–101 (1960).

Glassman, A.H., Hurwic, M.J. and Perel, J.M., Plasma binding of imipramine and clinical outcome. *American Journal of Psychiatry* 130, 1367–1369 (1973).

Gram, L.F., Metabolism of tricyclic antidepressants: a review. *Danish Medical Bulletin*, 21, 218–231 (1974).

Gram, L.F., Plasma level monitoring of tricyclic antidepressant therapy. *Clinical Pharmacokinetics* 2, 237–251 (1977a).

Gram, L.F., Factors influencing the metabolism of tricyclic antidepressants: studies on interaction and first pass elimination. *Danish Medical Bulletin* 24, 81–89 (1977b).

Gram, L.F., Reisby, N., Ibsen, J., Nagy, A., Dencker, S.F., Bech, P., Petersen, G.O., and Christiansen, J., Plasma levels and antidepressive effect of imipramine. *Clinical Pharmacology and Therapeutics* 19, 318–324 (1977).

Gurney, C., Roth, M., Garside, R.F., Kerr, T.A. and Schapira, K., Studies in the classification of affective disorders: the relationship between anxiety state and depressive illness. *British Journal of Psychiatry* 121, 162–166 (1972).

Hamilton, M., Rating scales in depression. In: *Depressive illness: Diagnosis, Assessment, Treatment*. Ed., Kielholz, Berne, 1972, pp. 100–107.

Hollister, L., Clinical use of psychotherapeutic drugs II: antidepressants and antianxiety drugs and special problems in the use of psychotherapeutic drugs. *Drugs* 4, 361–410 (1972).

Hollister, L., *Clinical Use of Psychotherapeutic Drugs*, 102–103, Springfield, Jil., 1973.

Kragh-Sørensen, P., Borgå, O., Garle, M., Hansen, L.B., Hansen, C.E., Hvidberg, E.F., Lassen, N. -E. and Sjöqvist, F., Effect of simultaneous treatment with low doses of perphenazine on plasma and urine concentrations of nortriptyline and 10-hydroxynortriptyline. *European Journal of Clinical Pharmacology* 11 479–483 (1977).

Kragh-Sørensen, P., Hansen, C.E. and Aasberg, M., Plasma nortriptyline levels in endogenous depression *Lancet* 1, 113–115 (1973).

Kragh-Sørensen, P., Hansen, C.E., Baastrup, P.C. and Hvidberg, E.F., Self-inhibiting action of nortriptyline's antidepressive effect at high plasma levels. *Psychopharmacologia* 45, 305–316 (1976).

Kragh-Sørensen, P., Hansen, C.E., Larsen, N. -E., Naestoft, J. and Hvidberg, E.F., Long-term treatment of endogenous depression with nortriptyline with control of plasma levels. *Psychological Medicine* 4, 174–180 (1974).

Kragh-Sørensen, P., Hvidberg, E.F., Hansen, C.E. and Baastrup, P.C., Therapeutic control of plasma concentrations and long-term effect of nortriptyline in recurrent affective disorders. *Pharmako. Psychiat.* 9, 178–182 (1976b).

Kragh-Sørensen, P., Jensen, K. and Klitgaard, N.A., "Single and multiple dose kinetics of doxepin in man: clinical application." Paper read at VI World Congress of Psychiatry, Honolulu, August 1977.

Kupfer, P.J., Hanin, J., Spiker, D.G., Grau, T. and Coble, P., Amitriptyline plasma levels and clinical response in primary depression. *Clinical Pharmacology and Therapeutics* 22, 904–911 (1977).

Montgomery, S.A., and Braithwaite, R.A., "The relationship between plasma concentration of amitriptyline and therapeutic response." Paper read at British Association of Psychopharmacology meeting, London, July 1975.

Montgomery, S.A., Braithwaite, R.A. and Crammer, J.L., Routine nortriptyline levels in treatment of depression. *British Medical Journal* 166–167 (1977).

Montgomery, S.A., Braithwaite, R.A., Dawlings, S. and McAuley, R., High plasma nortriptyline levels in the treatment of depression. *Clinical Pharmacology and Therapeutics* 23, 309–314 (1978).

Moody, J.P., Whyte, S.F., McDonald, A.J. and Naylor, G.J., Pharmacokinetic aspects of protriptyline plasma levels. *European Journal of Clinical Pharmacology* 11, 51–56 (1977).

Morris, J.B. and Beck, A.T., The efficacy of antidepressant drugs: a review of research (1958–1972). *Archives of General Psychiatry* 30, 667–674 (1974).

Pöldinger, W., Die Dosierung als ein wesentlicher Faktor der psychiatrischen Pharmakotherapie unter besonderer Berücksichtigung einer Kombination von Thiopropazat und Chlorphencyclan. In: *Proceedings of the Third Meeting of the Collegium Internationale Neuropsychopharmacologicum, Munich, 1963*. Eds., Bradley, P.B., Flügel, F. and Hoch, P.H., Amsterdam, 1964.

Reisby, N.,Gram, L.F., Bech, P., Nagy, A., Pedersen, G.O., Ortmann J., Ibsen, J., Dencker, S.F., Jacobsen, O., Krantwald, O., Søndergård, J. and Christiansen, J., Imipramine: clinical effects and pharmacokinetic variability. *Psychopharmacology* 54, 263–272 (1977).

Sjöqvist, F., A pharmacokinetic approach to the treatment of depression. *International Pharmacopsychiatry* 6, 147–169 (1971).

Sjöqvist, F., Hammar, W., Borgå, O. and Azarnoff, D.L., Pharmacological significance of the plasma level of monomethylated tricyclic antidepressants. In: *The Present Status of Psychotropic Drugs*. Ed., Cerletti, Amsterdam, 1969, pp. 128–136.

Sørensen, B., Kragh-Sørensen, P., Larsen, N. -E. and Hvidberg. E.F., The practical significance of nortriptyline plasma control. *Psychopharmacology* 59, 35–39 (1978).

Ziegler, V.E., Clayton, P.J., Taylor, J.R., Co, B.T., Biggs, J.T., Nortriptyline plasma levels and therapeutic response. *Clinical Pharmacology and Therapeutics* 20, 458–463 (1976).

Ziegler, V.E., Co, B.T., Taylor, J.R. and Biggs, J.T., Amitriptyline plasma levels and therapeutic response. *Clinical Pharmacology and Therapeutics* 19, 795–801 (1976).

8. COUMARIN ANTICOAGULANTS

M. L'E. ORME AND A.M. BRECKENRIDGE

Coumarin anticoagulants differ from most of the drugs discussed in this symposium volume in that, unlike tricyclic antidepressant or anticonvulsant drugs, their pharmacological and thus therapeutic effect can be accurately monitored. Whether the Thrombotest or the prothrombin time is measured the result is quickly, easily, and accurately obtained. Thus the measurement of plasma concentrations of coumarin anticoagulants is of little relevance in most clinical situations. There are however a few situations in which knowledge of the plasma coumarin concentration is of value.

There are four commonly used coumarin anticoagulants and their utilization varies from country to country. In the United Kingdom and Norway warfarin has now become the oral anticoagulant of choice, while in Sweden dicoumarol was until recently the most widely used anticoagulant although its use has now been officially discouraged because of its poor absorption and dose-dependent kinetics. In the Netherlands, phenprocoumon and acenocoumarol are the most popular. The important properties of these coumarin anticoagulants are shown in table 1. They all inhibit the synthesis of the vitamin-K-dependent clotting factors II, VII, IX and X. The supposed mechanism for this is shown in fig. 1. The coumarin anticoagulants are thought to work by inhibiting the reduction of vitamin-K epoxide back to vitamin K (Bell and Matschiner 1972) and studies with ^{3}H-vitamin K show an accumulation of vitamin-K epoxide in the plasma of patients being treated with warfarin (Shearer et al. 1977).

PLASMA COUMARIN ASSAYS

Several assay methods have been developed for the measurement of most coumarin anticoagulants in plasma. Most experience has been obtained with warfarin and thus this review will principally concern this drug. The early assays for the measurement of warfarin in plasma used either spectrophotometry (O'Reilly et al. 1962) or spectrofluorometry (Corn and Berberich 1967). While they were simple to perform they lacked sensitivity and in some cases were nonspecific since warfarin metabolites were also measured. A later adaption of the spectrofluorometric assay improved the measurement by introducing a thin-layer chromatography step which made the assay

Table 1. Characteristics of coumarin anticoagulants.

Anticoagulant	Peak prothrombin effect (h)	Duration of effect (days)	Plasma half-life (h)
Warfarin	36–60	4–5	25–60
Acenocoumarol	36–48	1.5–2	6–9
Phenprocoumon	48–72	7–14	120–180
Dicoumarol	36–48	5–6	60–100 (dose-dependent)

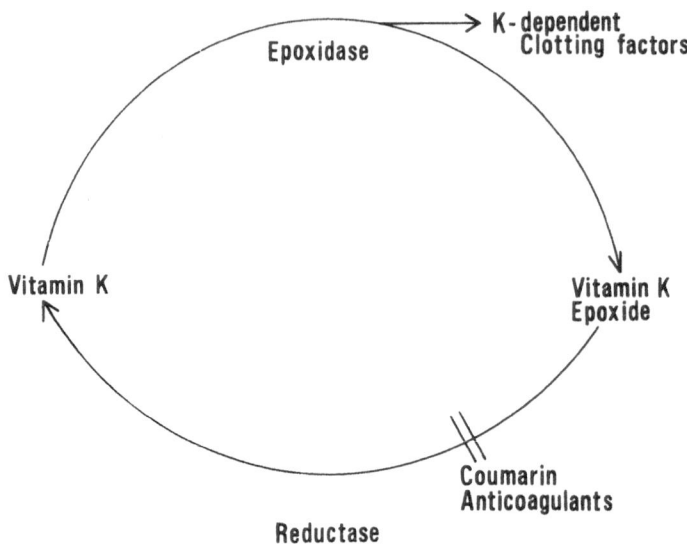

Figure 1. The suggested mode of action of oral anticoagulants on vitamin K.

specific for warfarin at the same time making it more tedious to perform (Lewis et al. 1970).

In our laboratory we use a modified gas liquid chromatographic assay (Kaiser and Martin 1974) which is both specific for warfarin and sensitive to 50 μg warfarin/l plasma. This method again has the disadvantage of being time-consuming but enables detailed pharmacokinetic studies to be undertaken if necessary. High-pressure liquid chromatographic assays have been developed (Fasco et al. 1977) and such assays may enable some of the metabolites of warfarin to be quantitated at the same time. Similar assays exist for the other coumarin anticoagulants (van Haelen-Fastré and van Haelen 1976). For phenprocoumon and acenocoumarol fluoridensitometric procedures have been described (de Wolff and van Kempen 1976; van Kempen et al. 1978). It is possible that in the future immunoassays will be developed that will make the measurement of plasma concentrations of these drugs both simpler and more sensitive.

PLASMA WARFARIN CONCENTRATIONS

In patients optimally controlled on long-term therapy with warfarin, we have a wide range in the plasma warfarin concentration (Breckenridge and Orme 1973). This is in part due to inter-individual variations in the pharmacokinetics of warfarin. There are also inter-individual differences in tissue sensitivity. In 23 patients, each of whom had been taking warfarin for at least three months, and each of whom had the same degree of anticoagulant control (Thrombotest 5–8 percent), the steady-state plasma warfarin concentration varied between 0.6 and 3.1 mg/l (Breckenridge and Orme 1973) representing a fivefold inter-individual difference.

COMPLIANCE

It is occasionally of value to measure the plasma warfarin concentration in patients who show very erratic anticoagulant control. Estimation of the prothrombin time will usually indicate that the patient is not adhering to the therapeutic regime and in only rare cases will measurement of the plasma warfarin add much to the management of the patient.

COVERT ANTICOAGULANT INGESTION

Covert anticoagulant ingestion can be a baffling diagnostic problem and coumarin anticoagulants can be used for a variety of unexpected ends. They have been used to commit suicide or murder and to procure abortion but the more usual form is to create factitious disease. Such patients have often been treated with oral anticoagulants in the past, may have a psychiatric history, or may be either doctors or nurses with access to the drug. Patients have frequently been extensively investigated in the haematology laboratory for unexplained bleeding or bruising before the possibility of anticoagulant ingestion is considered. The analysis of plasma for the presence of an anticoagulant; using a specific assay method, will often provide the answer to this problem. O'Reilly and Aggeler (1976) described 25 patients who presented with this condition and reviewed the literature of a further 48 cases. Patients may go to extreme lengths to conceal the true diagnosis from their physician and opinion is divided as to their further management. Psychiatric treatment is not always helpful and it may be unwise to reveal to the patient

that the true cause of their "illness" is known, since they may then resort
to the ingestion of drugs that are more difficult to detect. Bleeding and
bruising may be reversed by an injection of vitamin K.

PLASMA WARFARIN CONCENTRATIONS IN BREAST MILK

Recently we have used a gas liquid chromatographic assay for warfarin to
examine breast milk for warfarin. It has been stated as recently as 1976
(Verstraete and Verwilghen 1976) that warfarin is excreted in human breast
milk and that breast-feeding is thus contra-indicated. This information has
been based on nonspecific assay methods for warfarin which almost certainly measured warfarin metabolites (which are inactive) in the breast milk.
In twelve women, we were unable to detect warfarin in breast milk or in
the plasma of six of their infants, even at concentrations as low as $25 \mu g/l$
(Orme et al. 1977). Thus mothers on long-term therapy with warfarin can
breast-feed their infants without harm to the child.

PLASMA WARFARIN CONCENTRATION AND THERAPEUTIC EFFECT

The pharmacological effect of warfarin and the other coumarin anticoagulants does not correspond in time to the peak plasma concentration
of drug (see table 1). Nagashima et al. (1969) showed that the rate of synthesis
(R_{syn}) of the prothrombin complex did relate to plasma warfarin concentration, where

$$R_{net} = R_{syn} - R_{deg},$$

R_{net} being the net change of prothrombin time or Thrombotest per time
interval (usually six to twelve hours). R_{deg} is the rate of degradation of the
prothrombin complex activity and is measured as the rate constant for the
decay of prothrombin complex activity after a single dose of warfarin that
completely inhibits the synthesis of the vitamin-K-dependent clotting
factors. The rate of synthesis of the prothrombin complex activity per unit
time can then be measured during the recovery phase of prothrombin complex activity after the same single dose of warfarin. The plasma warfarin
concentration can then be plotted against the rate of clotting factor synthesis
as shown in fig. 2.

Warfarin, whose chemical structure is shown in fig. 3, possesses an
asymmetric carbon atom (starred) and thus warfarin can exist in two
optically active forms, R(+) warfarin and S(−) warfarin. In all species so far
studied S(−) warfarin is more potent than R(+) warfarin and this is illustrated in fig. 2. (Breckenridge and Orme 1972). At any given plasma con-

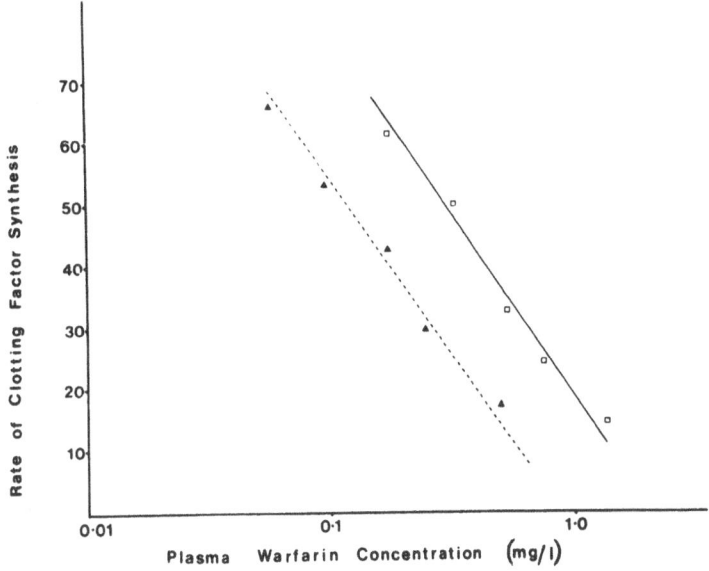

Figure 2. The rate of clotting factor synthesis (percent per twelve hours) plotted against the logarithmic value of the plasma warfarin concentration. Broken line: S(−) warfarin; continuous line R(+) warfarin.

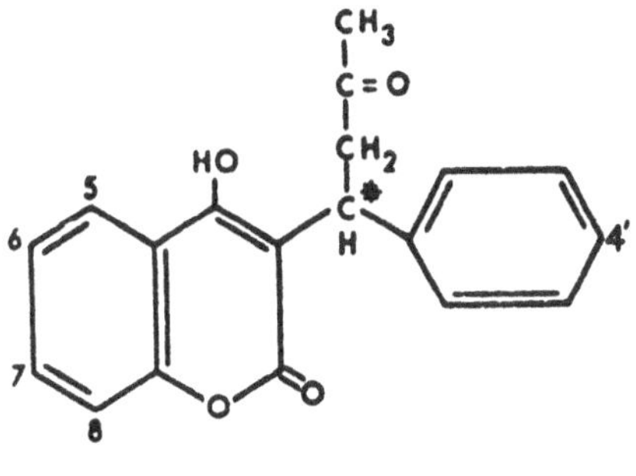

Figure 3. Chemical structure of warfarin.

centration of warfarin, S(−) warfarin produces a greater inhibition of clotting factor synthesis than R(+) warfarin. These enantiomers of warfarin also differ in other properties. In man S(−) warfarin has a shorter plasma half-life than R(+) warfarin, and the main metabolite of S(−) warfarin is 7-hydroxy warfarin while the main metabolite of R(+) warfarin is a reduction product, warfarin alcohol (Lewis et al. 1974). Phenprocoumon has also been shown to have two optically active enantiomers, S-phenprocoumon being more potent than R-phenprocoumon (Jähnchen et al. 1976).

WARFARIN RESISTANCE

Although the dose of warfarin needed for optimum anticoagulant control usually lies in the range 2–15 mg/day, occasional patients need considerably higher doses of warfarin to achieve this. In most of these cases this resistance to the therapeutic effects of warfarin is more apparent than real, and is due to failure of the patient to take the tablets regularly. Hereditary resistance to oral anticoagulants was first described by O'Reilly et al. (1964). In a patient who required 145 mg of warfarin per day to achieve anticoagulant control, the plasma warfarin concentration was commensurately elevated (55 mg/l), and no differences could be shown in the absorption, distribution or metabolism of warfarin compared to normal volunteers. O'Reilly (1969) described a second family with warfarin resistance. The daily dose needed was between 75 and 80 mg and eighteen of forty family members were resistant to large doses of warfarin. The genetic data indicated a dominant expression of a single gene located on an autosomal chromosome. These patients are also very sensitive to vitamin K. Patients are frequently referred to us because of resistance to the hypoprothrombinaemic effect of warfarin and measurement of the plasma warfarin concentration is of considerable help in the investigation of these problems. One such patient was taking 180 to 200 mg warfarin per day and was injected with this dose to ensure absorption. Plasma warfarin concentrations however were low (2.2 mg/l) in contrast to the patients described by O'Reilly (1969). After further questioning, the patient admitted taking a mixture of secobarbital and amobarbital (Tuinal®) prescribed for her sister. The patient ceased taking the barbiturate mixture and over the succeeding four months the daily warfarin requirement fell to 15 mg/day (see Breckenridge and Orme 1973). In this case microsomal enzyme induction by barbiturates was responsible for the resistance to warfarin.

DRUG INTERACTIONS WITH WARFARIN

The example just described illustrates a major change in warfarin metabolism that may occur as a result of a drug interaction. Measurement of the plasma warfarin concentration is of value in the understanding of the mechanism of such drug interactions. An example of such a study is shown in fig. 4. In this study the dose of warfarin is kept constant at 6 mg/day, a dose that is known in this patient to produce optimal anticoagulant control. During the initial period the plasma warfarin concentration is stable at about 1.3 mg/l but after the administration of phenazone in a dose of 600 mg/day there is a progressive loss of anticoagulant control and a fall in the plasma

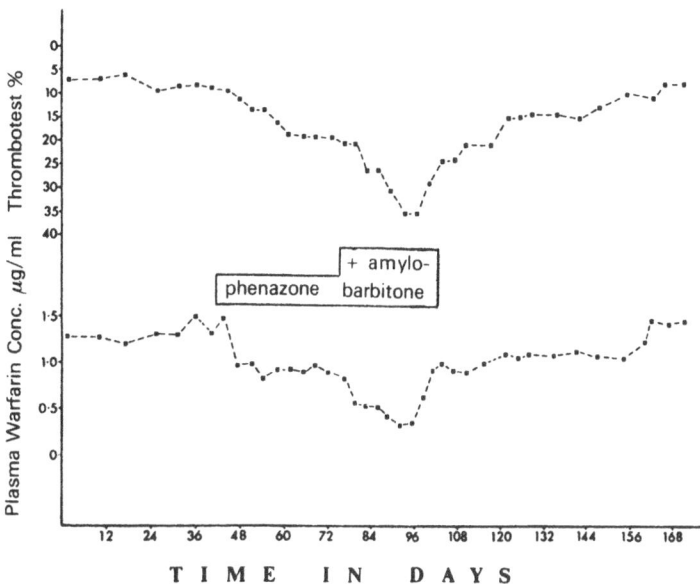

Figure 4. Plasma warfarin concentrations and Thrombotest values in a patient given 6 mg warfarin for 170 days before, during and after the administration of phenazone 600 mg/day for 30 days followed by phenazone 600 mg/day plus amylobarbitone 200 mg nightly for 21 days.

warfarin concentration to about 0.8 mg/l over the succeeding three weeks. After a period of relative stability during the next ten days, the addition of amylobarbitone 200 mg at night to the phenazone treatment causes a further loss of anticoagulant effect due to a fall in the plasma warfarin concentration to about 0.4 mg/l. This datum provides indirect evidence of an increased rate of warfarin metabolism as the explanation of the loss of anticoagulant effect.

Measurement of plasma warfarin concentrations is important in studying the effect of an agent which displaces warfarin from sites of protein binding. Displaced warfarin gives rise to an enhanced pharmacological effect but is also more available for metabolism within the liver. The interaction between phenylbutazone and warfarin has always been attributed to this mechanism, where increased free warfarin concentrations in plasma following displacement lead to an enhanced hypoprothrombinaemic effect. Recent studies have shown that the real mechanism is considerably more complicated than this original explanation. In these studies, R(+) warfarin and S(−) warfarin were administered separately to volunteers before and during phenylbutazone therapy. The elimination of S(−) warfarin, the more potent enantiomer, was reduced from 2.7 to 1.4 percent per hour while the elimination of R(+) warfarin was increased from 1.2 to 2.3 percent per hour. Thus the overall elimination of racemic warfarin was unchanged by phenylbutazone but the hypoprothrombinaemic effect was enhanced because the plasma concentration of the more potent enantiomer, S(−) warfarin, was increased by phenylbutazone (Lewis et al. 1974). Studies of drug interactions with oral anticoagulant drugs will be improved further when it becomes possible to measure plasma concentrations of both warfarin enantiomers after administration of the racemic mixture to man.

CONCLUSIONS

Plasma concentrations of coumarin anticoagulants are not of routine value because the therapeutic effect of the drugs themselves is so easily measured. Measurement of plasma concentrations can be of value in the management of patients who may have ingested anticoagulants surreptitiously or in whom compliance may be a problem. Knowledge of the plasma concentration may also be of value in patients who appear to be resistant to the effects of oral anticoagulants and in the investigation of drug interactions with oral anticoagulants.

REFERENCES

Bell, R.G. and Matschiner, J.T., Warfarin and the inhibition of vitamin K activity by an oxide metabolite. *Nature* 237, 32–33 (1972).
Breckenridge, A.M. and Orme, M.L'E., The plasma half lives and the pharmacological effect of the enantiomers of Warfarin in rats. *Life Sciences* 2, 2, 337–345 (1972).
Breckenridge, A.M. and Orme, M.L'E., Measurement of plasma Warfarin concentrations in clinical practice. In: *Biological Effects of Drugs in Relation to Their Plasma Concentrations*. Ed., Davies, D.S., and Prichard, B.N.C., London, 1973, pp. 143–154.
Corn, M. and Berberich, R., Rapid fluorometric assay for Warfarin. *Clin. Chemistry* 13, 126–131 (1967).
Fasco, M.J., Piper, L.J. and Kaminsky, L.S., Biochemical applications of a quantitative high-pressure liquid chromatographic assay of Warfarin and its metabolites. *J. Chromatography* 131, 365–373 (1977).
Jähnchen, E., Meinertz, T., Gilfrich, H.J., Groth, U. and Martini, A., The enantiomers of phenprocoumon: pharmacodynamic and pharmacokinetic studies. *Clin. Pharm. Ther.* 20, 342–349 (1976).
Kaiser, D.G. and Martin, R.S., GLC determination of Warfarin in human plasma. *J. Pharm. Sci.* 10, 1579–1583 (1974).
Van Kempen, G.M.J., Koot-Gronsveld, E.A.M. and de Wolff, F.A., Quantitative and qualitative analysis of the anticoagulant acenocoumarol in human plasma. *J. Chromatog. Biomed. Appl.* 145, 332–335 (1978).
Lewis, R.J., Ilnicki, L.P. and Carlstrom, M.; The assay of Warfarin in plasma or stool. *Biochem. Medicine* 4, 376–382 (1970).
Lewis, R.J., Trager, W.F., Chan, K.K., Breckenridge, A.M., Orme, M.L'E. Roland, M. and Schary, W., Warfarin: stereochemical aspects of its metabolism and the interaction with Phenylbutazone. *J. Clin. Invest.* 53, 1607–1617 (1974).

Nagashima, R., O'Reilly, R.A. and Levy, G., Kinetics of pharmacological effects in man: the anticoagulant action of Warfarin. *Clin. Pharm. Ther.* 10, 22–35 (1969).

O'Reilly, R.A., The second reported kindred with hereditary resistance to oral anticoagulant drugs. *New Eng. J. Med.* 282, 1448–1452 (1969).

O'Reilly, R.A. and Aggeler, P.M., Covert anticoagulant ingestion: study of 25 patients and review of world literature. *Medicine* 55, 389–399 (1976).

O'Reilly, R.A., Aggeler, P.M., Hoag, M.S. and Leong, L., Studies on the coumarin anticoagulants: the assay of Warfarin and its biological application. *Thrombosis et Diathesis Haemorrhagica* 8, 82–95 (1962).

O'Reilly, R.A., Aggeler, P.M., Hoag, M.S. and Leong, L., Hereditary transmission of exceptional resistance to coumarin anticoagulant drugs. *New Eng. J. Med.* 271, 809–815 (1964).

Orme, M.L'E., Lewis, P.J., M., de Swiet, Serlin, M.J., Sibeon, R., Baty, J.D. and Breckenridge, A.M., May mothers given Warfarin breast feed their infants? *Brit. Med. J.* 1, 1564–1565 (1977).

Shearer, M.J., McBurney, A., Breckenridge, A.M. and Barkhan, P., Effect of Warfarin on the metabolism of Phylloquinone (vitamin K_1): dose-response relationships in man. *Clin. Sci. Mol. Medicine* 52, 621–630 (1977).

Van Haelen-Fastré, R., and van Haelen, M., High performance liquid and thin-layer chromatography of coumarin anticoagulants and their degradation products. *J. Chromatography* 129, 397–402 (1976).

Verstraete, M. and Verwilghen, R., Haematological disorders. In: *Drug Therapy*. Ed., Avery, G.S., Sydney, 1976, pp. 661–716.

De Wolff, F.A. and van Kempen, G.M.J., Determination of phenprocoumon, an anticoagulant, in human plasma. *Clin. Chem.* 22, 1575–1578 (1976).

PART IIB

APPLICATIONS TO SPECIFIC DRUGS

9. ANTIMICROBIAL DRUGS

H. MATTIE

The determination of plasma concentrations of antimicrobial drugs has a relatively long history. There are several reasons for this, one being that these determinations are easy to perform with microbiological procedures. These have played an important role in the development of antibiotics from the very beginning. When penicillin was available as an impure substance it was necessary to assess the antibacterial activity of the product against a standard in a bioassay procedure, and to express the strength in so-called Oxford units. Penicillin dosage is still expressed as units instead of milligrams, notwithstanding the fact that benzylpenicillin has been available as a pure substance for a long time. The same principle was applied in the early forties for the assay of concentrations of penicillin in body fluids, and is still used today. However, the methods in those early days were rather crude, and cumbersome at the same time.

MICROBIOLOGICAL METHOD

Today most microbiological methods go back to the standard work of Grove and Randall (1955), a book that has not been reprinted for more than twenty years. The most frequently employed method is the so called agar diffusion technique. In this technique a bacterial culture is mixed with agar and then poured out in a petri dish. After cooling a thin smooth layer is formed in which bacteria can grow under incubation at 30 or 37°C; after incubation for eighteen hours the plate has an opaque appearance. Before incubation small holes are cut in the plate in each of which a small volume of fluid can be placed, containing the antibiotic. This diffuses into the agar around the hole, so that bacterial growth is inhibited. Over a certain range of concentrations the diameter of the growth inhibition zone is practically linearly dependent on the logarithm of the concentrations. Therefore a series of twofold dilutions is made of a standard solution, and the zone diameters are plotted against the dilution, giving a fairly straight standard line. The zone diameter around the unknown sample is then interpolated on this line and the concentration can be read easily if a logarithmic scale is used for the standard dilutions.

Sensitivity, precision and accuracy
The sensitivity of this microbiological method is nearly always more than sufficient for clinical practice. This is not quite unexpected, because anti-bacterial activity is the effect to be measured in the bioassay, and it is the antibacterial activity that is relevant for serum concentrations. Nevertheless, the test organism has to be more sensitive than the pathogenic microorgan-ism, because of the small sample volumes involved. In other words, it is seldom feasible to use the pathogen isolated from a patient as a test organ-ism. In most instances, however, this is irrelevant.

The precision of the method is better than is often taken for granted by people who think that newer, more expensive, equipment is indispensable for reliable results. In bioassays, the precision of the results depends on two characteristics: the slope of the regression line of zone diameters on con-centrations, and the variation of zone diameters around the regression line. In microbiological assays the most important variable for determining the precision is most often the slope, and this depends mainly on the test organism. In this respect penicillins can be measured more precisely than, for example, chloramphenicol or gentamicin. We have modified the method described above, so as to be able to assess the precision in each individual determination (Mattie et al. 1973). A classical four-point bioassay is per-formed, with duplicates of each point. Two dilutions of the standard and two of the unknown are chosen, producing zone diameters preferably between 16 and 24 mm, because in this range reproducibility is optimal (fig. 1). By this method it is possible to calculate the standard deviation with-in the assay. For penicillins this is mostly less than 5 percent, for gentamicin it may amount to 10 or 11 percent. Ninety-five percent probability limits are

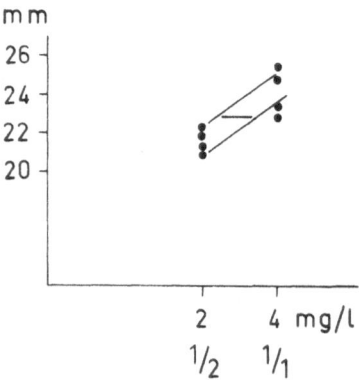

Figure 1. Example of a four-point bioassay of an antibiotic.

therefore about ± 20 percent for gentamicin. Even the latter value compares favourably with many more advanced techniques used for this or other kinds of drugs. The most debatable characteristic is, however, the accuracy. One of the objections often heard is that in this method only antibacterial activity is measured and not the drug itself. This is not a relevant objection: with no other method is the drug itself measured, but only a certain quantitative value that is related to it: e.g. radioactivity in radioimmunoassay, a peak in a gas chromatogram, an extinction in spectrophotometry. Therefore, in this respect, there is no fundamental difference between microbiological and other methods. Still it has limitations of its own. Many test organisms are sensitive to many antibiotics, so when a patient is treated with a combination of antibiotics it is impossible to assess the concentration of a single one of them properly. It is sometimes argued that this is not so important, because one can determine the combined antibacterial activity. That is very doubtful reasoning however, because it is not the antibacterial activity against the test organism that interests the clinician. One could try the patients own pathogen as a test organism, but that is often impracticable, and moreover it should not be regarded as a bioassay, but as a kind of *in vitro* test of unproven value. One way out is the employment of a test organism that is sensitive to only one of the drugs of the combination, after excluding synergy of the combination against the test organism. Other devices are: adding of beta-lactamase to destroy penicillins or cephalosporins, or cellulose phosphate to inactivate aminoglycosides (Stevens and Young 1977). This may be a warning how important it is that the laboratory should have full information on the use of other antibiotics, to avoid erroneous results.

Metabolites pose greater problems. Of course the advantage of the method is that it is not sensitive to inactive metabolites. There are active metabolites however with an activity against the test organism that differs from that against the pathogen. A good example is cloxacillin: this anti-staphylococcal penicillin has two biologically active metabolites, the activity of which against some test organisms differs from that against *S. aureus* (Thijssen and Mattie 1976). In clinical practice this does not make much difference, as the concentration of the metabolites in plasma is only about ten percent. In severe renal failure however this percentage may increase to as much as forty percent. Not much is known about the role of active metabolites as a bias in the bioassay of other antibiotics. Probably they are not very important in the case of aminoglycosides because these drugs are scarcely metabolized.

Another source of bias is the following: in an ideal bioassay the standard is made identical to the sample, except of course for concentrations. For the determination of urinary concentrations this is practically impossible: no two urines are identical in composition. Therefore it is common practice to use a standard in water. A lucky circumstance is that urinary concentrations are so high that urine has to be much diluted to perform the assay. Nevertheless some precautions should be taken, e.g. for aminoglycosides the standard and the sample should have the same pH value. For serum or plasma samples a standard in pooled human serum is quite a good approximation, although in some patients there are important differences in serum composition, as for example in the conditions of hypalbuminaemia and uraemia. It is well known by now that the serum of uraemic patients contains a factor that changes protein binding of many antibiotics, most often diminishing it. Thus the two conditions mentioned pose the same problem for the determination of the concentrations. Protein binding, as a matter of fact, may slow down the diffusion of antibiotics into the surrounding agar, giving smaller zone diameters in this way. It does not do so in a simple way, and therefore it is certainly not warranted to imply that in this way the concentration of the unbound, active, drug is determined. As it is often impossible in clinical practice to use the patient's own serum to prepare a standard, the only possibility is to keep this in mind in interpreting results. However, since only the unbound drug is the active part of the concentration, the error in neglecting this problem is sometimes less severe than one might expect.

A last disadvantage of the microbiological determination of antibiotics is its slowness: inevitably it takes some time before bacterial growth is visible. The disadvantage is of less clinical importance than one might think, since it is rarely necessary to have quick results. It is possible however, even with biological methods, to have a preliminary result the same day.

For these reasons other methods have been developed, the advantages of which are naturally claimed by the originators. Some of those are partly biological, but require extra equipment: measurement of pH changes, or of bacterial ATP, to mention a few possibilities. The main advantage over the older biological methods is their rapidity. Chemical methods have been used for some chemotherapeutic drugs like sulfonamides, but for antibiotics they have never become popular. Of the newer methods high-pressure liquid chromatography seems to be the most promising. The investment is of course rather costly, and worthwile only when the demand is great. One should be aware of the rule that expensive investments can induce a greater demand which makes the cost per item less, but total costs higher. These methods have been dealt with in chapter 2.

CLINICAL INDICATIONS

The application has been used both in research and clinical practice. A peculiar circumstance should be mentioned in this respect. In most cases where diseases are treated with drugs one is dealing with a bilateral interaction between patient and drug. In infections however, a third party enters: the microorganism, giving rise to four more interactions. The microorganism is the target for the drug; moreover, it can be isolated easily from the patient and investigated *in vitro*. The effect of antibiotics on microorganisms *in vitro* has been studied extensively, and it has become good clinical practice to isolate the pathogen from a patient and to assess the susceptibility for antibiotics before making a rational choice for treatment. Of course this is a great advantage in the treatment of disease, but it has led to some over-simplification. First of all, the sensitivity of bacteria to antibiotics is nearly always expressed as the minimal inhibitory concentration (MIC) of the antibiotic. This is a well-defined effect, in terms of growth medium, temperature and time of exposure, but it is certainly not always the minimal effective concentration, even not *in vitro*. It is however not at all justified, without further experimental foundation, to put forward the MIC *in vitro* as the minimal effective concentration *in vivo* at the site of infection, where the interaction between microorganism and host plays such a predominant role (Mattie 1976; Mattie and Kunst 1976). Furthermore it is rather improbable that the concentration of the antibiotic at the site of infection is always equal to the plasma concentration, even if this is corrected for protein binding. Nevertheless, the ease with which serum concentrations of antibiotics can be determined has led to a vast amount of pharmacokinetic data that, carefully interpreted, can give a better understanding of this kind of drug. One aspect of the pharmacokinetics of antibiotics is certainly worthwhile mentioning, namely the data it can provide on the absorption after oral administration, not only in healthy volunteers, but especially in patients. Such data make one aware of the fact that in patients absorption of antibiotics is often more erratic than in healthy volunteers (Kunst and Mattie 1975).

In clinical practice the most important application of the determination of serum concentrations is to assess whether they are in the range that has been established as sufficient for the treatment of a particular disease, or as non-toxic. A good example is in the case of a young woman, with an underlying malignant disease, who had acquired a *Salmonella* osteomyelitis and was treated with oral ampicillin. When the clinical course of this treatment was not very satisfactory two things were done: the exact MIC of the microorganism was determined (which is not done normally), and the absorption was estimated by determining concentrations in a few well-chosen serum samples. The MIC showed us that the *Salmonella* was clearly less sensitive than expected on the basis of the experience with this group of microorganisms. The serum concentrations were well below those normally found. This led to the decision to treat the patient for a long period with ampicillin intravenously at higher dosages, with good result. The MIC was regarded in this instance as a relative instead of an absolute value, and as such it is indeed in our opinion more reliable. This kind of experience in the past has led us to earlier and more frequent determinations of serum concentrations. For different groups of antibiotics, for different routes of administration and for different diseases, the indications and the sampling times and the samples themselves are different.

Beta-lactam antibiotics

The β-lactam antibiotics, penicillins and cephalosporins, are characterized by a short to a very short half-life in plasma. Therefore, when they are administered intravenously at regular intervals, they do not accumulate. This holds also, more or less, for intramuscular injections in normal, well-vascularized muscle. This implies that there will not be much variation in plasma concentrations between patients, or in other words, in the relation between dose and concentration. Therefore, if the dose is that required, according to clinical experience, there is no need to determine serum concentrations. This may be different in those infections where a certain minimal concentration is regarded, rightly or wrongly, as necessary for a good clinical result. That is the case, for instance, in endocarditis and in meningitis. These diseases are treated with high doses at frequent intervals. The minimal concentration, just before the next administration, is regarded as an indicator for the total diffusion pressure of the drug into the not easily reached sites of infection involved. If regarded as insufficient, the dose may be increased, or the interval shortened. In some clinics a continuous infusion is preferred in those circumstances. It then becomes mandatory to check serum concentrations at regular intervals, although not too frequently. It so happens that in this mode of administration serum concentrations are not only influenced by the volume of distribution, but also to a great extent by the clearance. The latter is more difficult to estimate than the former, because it may vary considerably between patients. Once the proper infusion rate is established, corrections for changes in antibiotic clearance can be made easily because these are reflected largely by changes in creatinine concentrations. When changing from parenteral to oral administration it is often wise to check whether satisfactory concentrations are reached, because many penicillins are absorbed poorly after oral administration.

In this instance a pre-administration value is not sufficient, although it is the minimal concentration, its relation to the maximal or the mean plasma concentration is variable, due to differences in absorption rates. Indeed a slow and incomplete absorption may give rise to higher pre-administration concentrations than a rapid and complete one. Therefore another estimate should be made one or two hours before administration. If the difference is much less than expected from what is known of the half-life of the antibiotic, this is an indication that absorption is slow, and probably incomplete.

When rapid absorption may be expected, for instance with amoxicillin or cephalexin, and the interval is large, it is preferable to take the two samples somewhat earlier, e.g. three and four hours after administration. Since the penicillins and even the cephalosporins are relatively innocuous drugs it is not necessary to measure serum concentrations for reasons of toxicity; only if very high dosages are given in patients with severely impaired renal function may toxicity in the form of convulsions become apparent.

Aminoglycosides

Toxicity is the main reason for frequent estimates of aminoglycoside antibiotics. This kind of drug has a very low therapeutic index in infections with marginally sensitive microorganisms, like *Pseudomonas*. Ototoxicity is the most feared toxic manifestation of aminoglycosides because it is irreversible, while nephrotoxicity is nearly always completely reversible. Nephrotoxicity is possible concentration-dependent, but to monitor the patients for early signs it is probably better to follow the serum creatinine closely than to measure antibiotic concentrations. Impaired renal function however in itself gives rise to higher plasma concentrations, because these drugs are excreted practically exclusively by the kidney. In this way nephrotoxicity enhances the danger of ototoxicity, which in itself is probably very closely related to plasma concentrations and time of exposure. In patients with normal renal function who are treated for not longer than seven to ten days damage to the labyrinth will probably be very limited, at least when the maximal concentration does not exceed the limits that are generally considered as safe (25–30 mg/l for kanamycin and streptomycin; 8–10 mg/l for gentamicin and tobramycin). These maximal concentrations can be predicted fairly correctly by assuming that the volume of distribution is about 25 percent of the body weight, so there is indeed no need for very rapid serum determinations. But it is necessary to verify within one or two days whether the initial guess was right, and the dosage should be adjusted accordingly. When renal function is impaired correct dosage becomes more difficult, especially when rapid changes occur. The principles remain rather simple, because mean serum concentrations of the antibiotic will rise to the same extent as the creatinine clearance falls, but in practice some experience is helpful. Also nomograms or even computer programs may be useful, but they too should not be used without thought, and anyway they should always be verified by serum concentrations. It is a matter of opinion whether the abovementioned maximal limits are still safe in case of renal impairment; probably they are not. It is plausible that the total exposure of the inner ear depends just as much on the minimal concentrations. When absorption after injection is rapid, the total area under the serum concentration-time curve, or, the concentration-time product, is approximately equal to

$$\frac{C_{max} - C_{min}}{\ln C_{max} - \ln C_{min}}$$

per day, corresponding with the mean plasma concentration.

When this kind of toxic antibiotic is administered for a long time locally, e.g. neomycin orally in hepatic cirrhosis, it may be worthwhile to know how much of it is absorbed. Absorption should be absent, but it does occur sometimes, albeit slowly. The best estimate of absorption is then the total amount excreted in the urine, not the concentration itself, in 24 hours, this being better than serum concentrations, which are often too low to measure accurately.

In cases of renal impairment due to aminoglycosides it could be worthwhile following up urinary excretion for a long period, since it has been shown that in these cases the drug has become bound to the renal parenchyma. Unfortunately microbiological methods are too insensitive to detect residual antibiotic after some time lapse.

Other antimicrobial agents

Most other antibiotics are not so closely monitored during therapy. There are several reasons for that: sometimes because they are absorbed in a rather predictable way, like doxycyclin; sometimes because the infections are not so serious that the clinical result cannot be awaited, as is the case in for instance many urinary tract infections.

The only other important group is that of tuberculostatic drugs. Because treatment takes a long time before clinical results become conspicuous, and absorption is often erratic, serum concentrations should be measured at an early stage of treatment. The microbiological method to determine isoniazide is much slower than normal, because of the slow growing test organism, and a chemical method would be preferable.

Conclusion

In conclusion, for most antibiotics microbiological determinations are reliable, not very difficult to perform, and often of great help in the treatment of infections.

REFERENCES

Grove, D.C. and Randall, W.A., *Assay methods of antibiotics: A Laboratory Manual.* New York, 1955.

Kunst, M.W. and Mattie, H., Absorption of pivampicillin in postoperative patients *Antimicrob. Agents Chemother.* 8, 11–14 (1975).

Mattie, H., The *in vivo* significance of antibiotics in the tissues. *Chemotherapy* 4, 7–12 (1976).

Mattie, H. and Kunst, M.W., The *in vivo* significance of tissue concentration. *Infection* 4, suppl. 2, 164–167 (1976).

Mattie, H., Goslings, W.R.O. and Noach, E.L. Cloxacillin and nafcillin: serum binding and its relationship to antibacterial effect in mice. *J. of Inf. Dis.* 128, 2, 170–177 (1973).

Stevens, P. and Young, L.S., Simple methods for elimination of aminoglycosides from serum to permit bioassay of other antimicrobial agents. *Antimicrob. Agents Chemother.* 12, 2, 286–287 (1977).

Thijssen, H.H.W. and Mattie, H., Active metabolites of isoxazolylpenicillins in humans. *Antimicrob. Agents Chemother.* 10, 3, 441–446 (1976).

10. METHOTREXATE AND OTHER ANTINEOPLASTIC AGENTS

H.M. PINEDO AND P.M. WILKINSON

Assays for many drugs have made it possible to establish concentration ranges for their safe and therapeutically effective use. However, with the exception of methotrexate (MTX) and possibly adriamycin and cytosine arabinoside, drug schedules for antineo-plastic agents are at present based on empiric observations and such parameters as organ toxicity and clinical antitumor effectiveness are used as major guidelines. Correlations between drug level, therapeutic effectiveness and toxicity have been observed for MTX, whose activity can be determined directly, because this compound is only minimally metabolized. Most of the other antineo-plastic agents are converted to the active metabolite before they exert their effect. These active metabolites are formed in the liver cells or in other cells such as the target tumor cell itself. Nevertheless, assays of other anticancer agents have provided considerable information about their pharmacological para-meters and mechanism of action. Because of the unique place MTX occupies in this respect within the group of anticancer agents, this drug requires de-tailed discussion. It would be improper not to review the vast amount of data on experimental pharmacokinetics which initiated the rapid development of clinical pharmacokinetics.

METHOTREXATE

Experimental pharmacokinetics: effect of MTX on cultured cells
The antifolate MTX is a potent inhibitor of the enzyme dihydrofolate re-ductase, displaying stoichiometric binding to the mammalian enzyme at a pH of 6.1 and limited competitive substrate (Johns and Bertino 1973). A considerable amount of free intracellular MTX at least equalling dihydro-folate reductase levels is required to detect partial inhibition of DNA syn-thesis in L1210 mouse leukaemia cells *in vitro* and *in vivo* (Goldman 1974).

In our studies on the potential of L1210 cells to form colonies *in vitro* in a semi-solid medium containing dialysed foetal calf serum, colony forma-tion occurred at MTX concentrations of up to 10^{-6} M. The colonies grown in the presence of MTX were, however, significantly smaller than the control colonies. Our findings are in agreement with the findings of Sirotnak and Donsbach (1973, 1975) showing an *in vitro* requirement of 10^{-6}M MTX for

50 percent inhibition of ^{3}H-deoxyuridine incorporation. Thus, in both studies a considerably higher drug concentration was required to inhibit DNA synthesis *in vitro* than *in vivo*. The results of these experimental studies suggest that levels of the extracellular drug, which is in rapid exchange with the unbound intracellular drug, might be monitored as a measure of the free intracellular drug concentration, and thus might prove to have a relationship with the intracellular drug effect, which would be very useful. However, the relationship between extracellular and intracellular MTX concentrations has only been determined for a few experimental tumors and intestinal mucosa, and will have to be worked out for most tissues. Whereas tissue culture experiments have suggested that levels as high as 10^{-6} M are required to inhibit DNA synthesis, the threshold for the suppression of DNA synthesis *in vivo* appears to lie at 10^{-8} M for several tissues. At present we have no explanation for these findings. However, an imbalance of purine and pyrimidine nucleoside pools may partly explain this discrepancy. A 50 percent suppression of DNA synthesis *in vivo* at 10^{-8} M probably does not mean that DNA synthesis and cellular proliferation are totally inhibited at higher concentrations. These findings hold for murine and human bone marrow cells. The threshold concentration of MTX at which suppression of DNA synthesis is seen in gastro-intestinal mucosa lies at 5×10^{-9} M. In all probability the difference in the sensitivity of various tissues reflects differences in the permeability of the tissues to MTX.

Relationship of drug concentration and duration of exposure to cytotoxicity in vivo

The concept of a threshold level of free MTX for the inhibition of DNA synthesis led to the first meaningful interpretation of MTX pharmacokinetic data. The usefulness of the threshold was limited, because it provided no information about the relative importance of two factors, drug concentration and duration of exposure, in the genesis of cytotoxicity. In searching for a method to determine the importance of these two factors, we used constant infusion devices with different outputs (Pinedo et al. 1976a). Plasma concentrations of MTX were maintained at chosen levels with devices differing in size. The levels were measured by (1) the enzymatic assay, and (2) by the protein-binding assay. The mouse bone marrow was studied after exposure for various intervals. Under constant infusion of MTX, a maximum depletion of 70 percent of the nucleated bone marrow cells was observed at all concentrations between 10^{-8} and 10^{-5} M MTX. Maximum depletion was reached more rapidly at higher drug levels (Pinedo et al. 1977). For a given concentration of MTX, the fraction of surviving nucleated cells was a function of exposure until a plateau was reached. The nadir can probably be explained by the fact that cells are held up in the G_1-S interphase of the cell cycle.

At present we are studying the effects of the constant infusion of MTX on human bone marrow cells by culturing granulocyte precursor cells of bone marrow collected at various intervals during constant MTX infusion, in order to determine whether a similar self-limiting killing also occurs in the human bone marrow.

Effects of endogenous nucleosides on MTX activity*

We compared the potential of leucovorin and nucleosides in reversing, MTX toxicity for the granulocyte precursor cell (CFU-C) and for the L1210 mouse leukaemia cell. Both types of cell were cultured in the presence of the drugs in our semi-solid methylcellulose-based medium. Colony formation was assessed after seven days. The formation of 50-cell colonies was inhibited to 50 percent of control by 10^{-8} M MTX. Further increase in MTX concentration rapidly abolished colony formation by CFU-C (Pinedo et al. 1976b). Toxicity of 10^{-7} M MTX was completely reversed by equimolar concentrations of leucovorin, but at higher MTX concentrations, more leucovorin was required for the same effect. Whereas 10^{-5} M MTX was reversed by 10^{-3} M leucovorin, reversal of the toxic effect of 10^{-4} M MTX by 10^{-3} M leucovorin was not observed. In contrast to the reversal by leucovorin, toxicity of all MTX concentrations up to 10^{-4} M was completely prevented by 10^{-5} M thymidine combined with 10^{-5} M adenosine, inosine or hypoxanthine. Singly or at lower concentrations, nucleosides were ineffective. Thus, while leucovorin reversed the MTX toxicity to CFU-C competitively, reversal by nucleosides was non-competitive. In addition to these findings a slight thymidine toxicity at 10^{-4} M was observed and was total at 10^{-3} M.

Similar studies with L1210 mouse leukaemia cells gave quite different results. The threshold of activity of MTX was again 10^{-8} M, but the number of colonies formed showed only a small difference with the number in the controls up to an MTX concentration of 10^{-6} M. The size of these colonies differed greatly. When the importance of the size became apparent, we made use of an image analyser computer to express the size of the colonies in each experiment. The main differences compared to the CFU-C behaviour were as follows:

1. Colonies of L1210 develop in the presence of MTX up to a concentration of 10^{-6} M, however the colony size decreased with increasing drug concentration, and the threshold of activity was the same as that in the CFU-C (10^{-8} M);

2. Unlike the findings with the CFU-Cs, it was impossible to prevent

*This work has been supported by the Netherlands Cancer Society (Koningin Wilhelmina Fonds)

MTX cytoxicity for the L1210 cells by adding these nucleosides in equimolar concentrations;

3. Thymidine toxicity for the L1210 cells appears at a concentration of 5×10^{-5} M, and is almost total at a concentration of 10^{-4} M.

Further studies are required to explain why the L1210 cell cannot be rescued by thymidine and a purine nucleoside. Our findings may explain Tattersall's observation on L1210-bearing mice that thymidine rescues normal tissues selectivity *in vivo* (Tattersall et al. 1975). Thus there are two possible explanations for the therapeutic effectiveness of the MTX-thymidine schedule in L1210-bearing mice: (1) L1210 cannot be rescued by nucleosides; and (2) thymidine is toxic at a level of 10^{-5} M and higher. We are presently trying to find out whether selective rescue of normal tissues can be obtained during constant combined infusion of MTX and thymidine into L1210-bearing mice. These studies are being carried out under continuous monitoring of the MTX and thymidine levels.

Clinical pharmacokinetics: conventional dose
Until recently, little attention has been paid to the pharmacokinetics of low-dose MTX in man. It has been shown that the threshold of MTX concentration at which DNA synthesis is inhibited in man is 10^{-8} M. This is identical to the threshold concentration in mice. Recently we performed a pharmacokinetic study in eight of twenty patients with advanced head and neck cancer who were being treated with MTX in a dose of 100 mg/m^2, repeated every two weeks. The response rate was 60 percent. This is similar to the highest reported remission rate (61 percent) obtained with 1-gram doses given over a 36 h period and followed by leucovorin rescue. Others reported rates as low as 18 percent with a similar high-dose regimen. We observed two complete and ten partial remissions.

There appear to exist great variations in the plasma half-lives in patients on our regimen. The mean of the first half-life was 7 min (range 1–10 min), of the second half-life 1.6 h (range 0.9–2.2 h) and of the third half-life 7.5 h (range 5.3–11.5 h). Peak serum levels varied from 3×10^{-5} M to 10^{-5} M. The 24-hour serum concentration varied from as much as 10^{-8} M to 10^{-7} M. There was no correlation between the creatinine clearance and the MTX clearance. The urine excretion of MTX was measured from 0–12 h, 12–24 h, 24–48 h and 48–72 h. Although several patients excreted eventually more than 70 percent of the drug during the first twelve hours and a cumulative amount of more than 90 percent there was a large range in the proportion of MTX being excreted during the first three days (37–98 percent, mean 75 percent). There is a clear correlation between urinary elimination (percentage of administered dose) and toxicity ($r = 0.70$, $p = 0.007$). The three main signs of toxicity were nausea, mild stomatitis and epiphora. There is also a negative correlation ($r = -0.70$, $p = 0.027$) between the intercept of the third phase and probability of success. Thus, it seems that adjustment of the dose in the individual may improve the response rate.

High dose

High-dose MTX regimens (200 mg/kg) with leucovorin rescue have produced good responses in metastatic osteosarcoma (Jaffe and Pead 1972) and have increased the relapse-free interval when used as adjuvant after the surgical excision of non-metastatic osteogenic sarcoma. The MTX is infused over a period of 6 h and is followed by leucovorin rescue. This treatment has the potential of life-threatening toxicity for the patient. Monitoring of the plasma MTX concentrations 48 h after the initiation of infusion can identify patients with high risk of toxicity (Stoller et al. 1977). Patients with a plasma concentration higher than 9×10^{-7}M at 48 h are considered to show a delayed excretion of the drug. Patients with plasma concentrations below this level will not develop any toxicity. If adequate precautions are taken, patients with normal creatinine clearance will not show a delayed excretion of the drug. These precautions include the administration of 80 mEq sodium bicarbonate/m^2/24 h during 2 days. Hydration should begin 12 h before the MTX infusion is started and should be continued for 48 h. In addition, the pH of each urine sample should be checked during the first 48 h after the start of the MTX infusion. The MTX infusion should not be applied until the urine pH is above 7. If the urine pH drops below 7, additional bicarbonate should be given. If these recommendations are taken into consideration, the drug elimination will be adequate, the patient will not suffer toxicity, and measurement of the plasma level is not absolutely required. However, in cases with a borderline creatinine clearance (60–80 ml/min), monitoring of the plasma level at 48 h after the MTX infusion is mandatory. High-dose infusion is contraindicated in patients with a lower creatinine clearance. When an elevated plasma MTX level is found at 48 h, the leucovorin dose should be increased from 12–30 mg/m^2 to 50–100 mg/m^2 every 6 h. The duration of leucovorin administration should also be prolonged. Alkalinization of the urine and forced diuresis should be continued. These measures will prevent serious toxicity. Daily measurements of MTX levels are necessary until the plasma concentration of the drug has dropped below the threshold of toxicity, which is 10^{-8}M.

It has recently been shown by Jacobs and Santicky (1977) that there is no need to start leucovorin rescue shortly after terminating the MTX infusion. The administration of leucovorin may be postponed for at least 18 h after terminating the MTX infusion. When the fact is taken into consideration that our *in vitro* experiments indicate that the toxicity of MTX concentrations above 10^{-6}M is quite difficult to rescue, Jacob's observations are better understood. The indicated doses of leucovorin give plasma concentrations up to about 10^{-6}M but not higher. These concentrations would be able to rescue MTX toxicity caused by 10^{-7}M. This raises the question whether the first three leucovorin doses used at present in high-dose MTX treatment are of any benefit. It seems more logical to delay the initiation of leucovorin rescue.

CNS pharmacology

In addition to the use of MTX in systemic chemotherapy when given by the intrathecal route, this drug is very useful in the prophylaxis and treatment of meningeal leukaemia. Pharmacokinetic studies have been undertaken because of the high frequency of serious complications observed with this form of therapy. The half-life of MTX after single doses of 6–12 mg/m^2 is about 12 h in non-toxic patients but is significantly higher in patients who show signs of neurotoxicity (Bleyer et al. 1973). It is advisable to check the level in the spinal fluid 48 h after the intrathecal injection. If the level of MTX is above 2×10^{-7}M, the risk that toxicity will develop during treatment is much higher and the dose should be adjusted during the next course.

Pharmacokinetics in patients with large third spaces

Finally, the risks of toxicity in patients with a large third space should be mentioned. The elimination of the drug after intravenous administration may be greatly prolonged due to its accumulation in the fluid followed by slow backflow to the blood. This phenomenon can cause serious toxicity to normal tissues. A 24-h plasma level will single out patients in danger.

CONCLUSIONS

The several indications to perform the methotrexate assay in a patient may be summarized as follows:
   1. In high-dose treatment: 48-h plasma level;
   2. In intrathecal therapy: 48-hour spinal fluid level;
   3. In therapy in patients with large third spaces; and
   4. Possibly in conventional-dose therapy in general: peak plasma level and elimination curve (further study necessary).

PRESENT STATE OF CLIINICAL PHARMACOKINETICS OF OTHER DRUGS

Many assays are available for most of the other antineoplastic agents, but these methods have not been introduced into clinical oncology on a routine basis. Pharmacokinetic data have been obtained for most of these drugs and have given more insight into their mode of action, the development of toxicity, and other pharmacological parameters.

Investigations on 5-fluorouracil in man have revealed peak plasma levels of 10^{-4}M to 10^{-3}M after an intravenous injection of 15 mg/kg. The half-life is 10–20 min. after which plasma levels fall within 3 h to levels below 10^{-8}M (Cohen and Brennan 1973). Since 5-fluorouracil has to be converted intracellularly to the active metabolite 5-FdUMP, it is hardly surprising that it is not really feasible to use the assay of the drug to improve treatment results or prevent toxicity.

A similar situation exists for the pyrimidine analogue cytosine arabinoside (ara-C), which has to be converted intracellularly to ara-CTP before it can exert its activity (Ho and Frei 1971). Here again no correlation has been found between the anti-tumor effect and the drug level. The drug level is highly dependent on the ratio of deoxycytidine kinase (which activates the drug to the nucleotide form) to cytidine deaminase (which inactivates the drug to uracil-arabinoside). Tumor cells with a low kinase level are less responsive to the drug than those with high levels of this enzyme.

The anthracycline antibiotic adriamycin is metabolized in the liver to several compounds, some showing an anti-tumor activity comparable to that of the parent drug (Benjamin et al. 1973). Thus, pharmacokinetic studies on adriamycin should be aimed at measuring the whole spectrum of active products as well. The usefulness of the assay for other antineoplastic agents remains to be determined by experimental studies.

REFERENCES

Benjamin, R.S., Riggs. C.E., Jr. and Bachur, N.R., Pharmacokinetics and metabolism of adriamycin in man. *Clin. Pharm. Ther.* 14, 592–600 (1973).

Bleyer, W.A., Drake, J.C. and Chabner, B.A., Neurotoxicity and elevated cerebro-spinal fluid methotrexate concentration in meningeal leukemia. *New Engl. J. Med.* 289, 770–773 (1973).

Cohen, J.I. and Brennan, P.B., GLC assay for 5-FU in biological fluids. *J. Pharm. Sci.* 62, 572–575 (1973).

Goldman, I.D., The mechanisms of action of methotrexate In: interaction with low-affinity intracellular site required for maximum inhibition of deoxyribonucleic acid synthesis in L-cell mouse fibroblasts. *Mol. Pharmacol.* 10, 257–274 (1974).

Ho, D.H.W., and Fei III, E., Clinical pharmacology of l-beta-D-arabino-furanosylcytosine. *Clin. Pharm. Ther.* 12, 944–954 (1971).

Jacobs, S.A. and Santicky, M.J., Phase I trial of high dose methotrexate with modified citrovorum factor rescue. *Cancer Treatment Rep.* 62, 397–399 (1978).

Jaffe, N. and Pead, D., Recent advances in the chemotherapy of metastatic osteogenic sarcoma. *Cancer* 30, 1627–1631 (1972).

Johns, D.G. and Bertino, J.R., Folate antagonists. *Cancer Medicine* Ed., Holland J.F. and Frei III, E., Philadelphia, 1973, pp. 739–754.

Pinedo, H.M., Zaharko, D.S. and Dedrick, R.L., Constant infusion of methotrexate in mice. *Cancer Treatment Rep.* 60, 889–893 (1976a).

Pinedo, H.M., Zaharko, D.S., Bull, J.M. and Chabner, B.A., The reversal of methotrexate cytotoxicity to mouse bone marrow cells by leucovorin and nucleosides. *Cancer Res.* 36, 4418–4424 (1976b).

Pinedo, H.M., Zaharko, D.S., Bull, J. and Chabner, B.A., The relative contribution of drug concentration and duration of mouse bone marrow toxicity during continuous methotrexate infusion. *Cancer Res.* 37, 445–450 (1977).

Sirotnak, F.M. and Donsbach, R.C., Differential cell permeability and the basis for selective activity of methotrexate during therapy of the L1210 leukemia. *Cancer Res.* 33, 1290–1294 (1973).

Sirotnak, F.M. and Donsbach, R.C., Further evidence of a basis of selective activity and relative responsiveness during antifolate therapy of murine tumors. *Cancer Res.* 35, 1737–1744 (1975).

Stoller, R.G., Hande, K.R., Jacobs, S.A., Rosenberg, S.A. and Chabner, B.A., Use of plasma pharmacokinetics to predict and prevent methotrexate toxicity. *New Engl. J. Med.* 297, 630–634 (1977).

Tattersall, M.H.N., Brown, B., and Frei III, E., The reversal of methotrexate toxicity with maintenance of antitumor effects. *Nature* 253, 198–200 (1975).

11. DIGOXIN

G.E. MAWER

The relationship between the cardiac response to digoxin and the serum drug concentration is not direct. The transient, high serum concentrations which result from rapid intravenous injection are not associated with cardiac toxicity (Bertler et al. 1974). Similarly the cardiac response does not parallel the serum concentration during the early peak which corresponds with absorption from the gut. The response seems rather to parallel the hypothetical concentration of digoxin in a deeper, tissue compartment (Reuning et al. 1973). On theoretical grounds the mean concentration in such a compartment equals the mean serum concentration. Empirically the 24-hour mean serum digoxin concentration in patients receiving a daily maintenance dose is approximately equal to the concentration in a sample taken six to eight hours after the dose (Dobbs, Rodgers et al. 1976). The concentration in samples taken earlier is difficult to interpret. Similarly it is difficult to assess the appropriateness of a new dosage schedule from serum concentration data obtained prematurely before the one or two weeks have elapsed which are necessary for the attainment of a steady state.

Doubt is expressed about the therapeutic benefit conferred by digoxin on the patient with cardiac failure who is in sinus rhythm. Bearing this in mind and striving "above all to do no harm" the physician will seldom wish to produce steady state mean serum digoxin concentrations above 2 μg/l (2.6 nmol/l). Smith and Haber (1970) found that 87 percent of their patients with digitalis-induced cardiac arrhythmias had serum digoxin concentrations at or above this level; conversely 90 percent of their patients without such arrhythmias had lower levels.

Amongst patients with atrial fibrillation who had been known to have a rapid ventricular rate, a group mean serum digoxin concentration of 1 μg/l (1.3 nmol/l) was associated with barely adequate control (Chamberlain et al. 1970). Redfors (1972) found an average concentration of 1.1 μg/l (1.3 nmol/l) immediately before the daily dose in a group of patients with atrial fibrillation receiving individually determined optimum doses. Thus a steady-state mean serum digoxin concentration of 1–2 μg/l (1.3–2.6 nmol/l) probably represents a reasonable target in a patient whose response to digoxin is not yet known.

The largest daily oral dose commonly required by adult patients to maintain such a concentration is 500 μg of a formulation with a high dissolution rate. This dose of Lanoxin produced mean steady-state serum concentrations of 1.1–1.8 μg/l in six healthy volunteers with normal kidney function – creatinine clearance 90–120 ml/min (Kongola et al. 1976). The same daily dose produced mean concentrations of 1.2–2.6 μg/l in a group of outpatients with uncontrolled atrial fibrillation who were selected on the basis of a high apparent dosage requirement (Kongola et al. 1977). Before steps were taken to encourage compliance however these patients had serum concentrations of half the quoted values. The author believes that compliance should be questioned when patients appear to need larger doses.

At the other extreme of dosage requirements are adult patients with severe impairment of kidney function (creatinine clearance < 5ml/min). There were a few such patients in the study of Dobbs, Mawer et al. (1976) and they attained therapeutic concentrations with the smallest practical daily dose of 62.5 μg. This dose is also appropriate for a small proportion of elderly patients. Kongola (unpublished observations) measured the steady state six-to-eight-hour serum digoxin concentrations of fifty patients in a geriatric unit who were aged from 60 to 96 years. Five patients only attained levels of 1 μg/l or more when receiving 62.5 μg/day.

The digoxin dosage requirements of the majority of adult patients lie between these two extremes and it is reasonable to ask which clinical attribute provides the best prospective guide to dosage needs. The creatinine clearance estimated from the nomogram of Kampmann et al. (1974) was the best guide in a teaching hospital population with a wide range of kidney function (Dobbs, Mawer et al. 1976). This population contained however a relatively high proportion of patients referred for advice on dosage adjustment and was therefore not representative of the total population of adult patients for whom digoxin is prescribed.

Dobbs, Rodgers et al. (1977) measured the steady-state serum digoxin concentrations in an unselected population of 86 outpatients attending a general medical clinic. Assuming a linear relationship between daily dose and steady-state serum concentration they calculated how much digoxin was necessary for a pre-dose concentration of approximately 1 μg/l. This was then rounded off to the nearest practical dose. No patients requiring as little as 62.5 μg/day were encountered and only 12 who required as much as 500 μg/day. Patients with severe renal impairment were not represented, the lowest creatinine clearance being 34 ml/min and the correlation between dosage requirements and creatinine clearance was relatively weak; less than 50 percent of the variation in dosage requirements could be accounted for on this basis. The authors concluded that dosage based on creatinine clearance was little better than the administration of a fixed dose to all patients as a means of producing desired serum concentrations.

The commonest dosage requirement was 250 μg/day (32 patients) which is also the commonest digoxin dose prescribed at the time of discharge from the hospital in which the author works. The next most commonly required doses were 375 μg (26 patients) and 187.5 μg (12 patients) per day. Thus about 80 percent of the patients would have been appropriately treated so far as mean steady-state serum digoxin concentration was concerned by one of three daily doses. The attainment of a desired concentration does not however ensure an appropriate clinical response.

On 91 occasions simultaneous measurements of resting ventricular rate and mean steady-state serum digoxin concentration were made in patients with atrial fibrillation. The ventricular rate was appropriate (60–100 beats/min) on 31 out of 48 occasions when the concentration was 1–2 μg/l but on 6 occasions the rate was too fast and on 11 occasions it was too slow. There was therefore a case for adjusting digoxin dosage on the grounds of inappropriate ventricular rate in about one third of the instances in which desired concentrations had been successfully achieved.

The attainment of a mean steady-state serum concentration of 1–2 μg/l equally does not ensure freedom from toxicity. Dobbs et al. (1977) found no clear relationship between subjective toxic features such as anorexia, nausea and diarrhoea and the serum concentration; one third of their patients (19 of 57) with serum concentrations of 1–1.8 μg/l showed these features and the same proportion (11 of 29) of those with higher concentrations (1.8–2.6 μg/l) was similarly affected.

Aronson et al. (1978) used multivariate analysis to assess the relationship between the serum digoxin concentration and the likelihood of unequivocal digoxin toxicity. High-risk factors were a serum digoxin concentration exceeding 3 μg/l, a serum potassium concentration outside the normal range, age above 60 years, dose above 6 μg/kg/day and a serum creatinine concentration above 150 μmol/l. They were not able to detect a relationship between digoxin-induced cardiac toxicity and serum concentration at levels below 3 μg/l. The provisional clinical diagnosis of digoxin toxicity is established by observing recovery after digoxin withdrawal. Only in the rare circumstances of very high mean serum digoxin concentration can the serum assay provide direct evidence of intoxication.

These observations have practical implications for patient management. The number of patients treated with digoxin is large, perhaps 300,000 in the United Kingdom alone (*Lancet* 1976), thus the routine use of digoxin radioimmunoassay as a check on the appropriateness of dosage would be very expensive and it is difficult to believe that this would be justified by a commensurate improvement in patient well-being. Cardiac response would remain the critical factor in the choice of dose. The range of dosage requirements in the adult population is not large and a given patient is very likely to be appropriately treated by one of three daily dosage rates. Probably the main reason for serum digoxin assay is the need to distinguish between insensitivity to digoxin and non-compliance in a patient who appears to need a dose which is disproportionately large for his level of kidney function.

CONCLUSIONS

1. The serum digoxin concentration of relevance to long-term therapy is probably the mean, steady-state value. An approximate estimate can be obtained from a single sample collected 6–8 h after the daily dose. The generally suitable concentration is 1–2 μg/l.

2. The daily oral dose of a rapidly dissolving formulation required to produce this concentration in adult patients varies over an eightfold range (62.5–500 μg/day) according to kidney function (creatinine clearance). The dosage requirement of most patients attending a general medical clinic however varies over a twofold range only (187.5–375 μg/day).

3. In an individual patient the cardiac effect of a mean serum concentration of 1–2 μg/l may be appropriate, excessive or inadequate and the likelihood of digoxin toxicity is largely determined by coincidental factors. Thus dosage adjustment is based chiefly on patient response and the therapeutic relevance of serum digoxin assays is limited.

REFERENCES

Aronson, J.K., Grahame-Smith, D.G. and Wigley, F.M., Monitoring digoxin therapy: the use of plasma digoxin concentration measurement in the diagnosis of digoxin toxicity. *Quarterly Journal of Medicine* 47, 111–122 (1978).
Bertler, A., Bergdahl, B. and Karlsson, E., Plasma digoxin concentrations after an intravenous loading dose. *Lancet* 2, 958 (1974).
Chamberlain, D.A., White, R.J., Howard, M.R. and Smith, T.W., Plasma digoxin concentrations in patients with atrial fibrillation. *British Medical Journal* 3, 429–432 (1970).
Dobbs, S.M., Mawer, G.E., Rodgers, E.M., Woodcock, B.G. and Lucas, S.B., Can digoxin dose be predicted? *British Journal of Clinical Pharmacology* 3, 231–237 (1976).
Dobbs, S.M., Rodgers, E.M., Mawer, G.E. and Kenyon, W.I., Serum digoxin concentrations. *British Journal of Clinical Pharmacology* 3, 674–676 (1976).
Dobbs, S.M., Rodgers, E.M., Kenyon, W.I., Livshin, D., Slater, E. and Godsmark, B., Digoxin prescribing in perspective. *British Journal of Clinical Pharmacology* 4, 327–335 (1977).
Kampmann, J., Siersbaek-Nielsen, K., Kristensen, M. and Mølholm Hansen, J., Rapid evaluation of creatinine clearance. *Acta Medica Scandinavica* 196, 517–520 (1974).
Kongola, G., Mawer, G.E. and Woodcock, B.G., Steady state pharmacokinetics of β-methyl digoxin and digoxin. *British Journal of Clinical Pharmacology* 3, 954 (1976).
Kongola, G.W.M., Coburn, P.R. and Mawer, G.E., Comparison of medigoxin and digoxin in patients with atrial fibrillation. *British Journal of Clinical Pharmacology* 4, 727 (1977).
Lancet, Editorial: foxglove saga. *Lancet* 2, 405 (1976).
Redfors, A., Plasma digoxin concentration: its relation to digoxin dosage and clinical effects in patients with atrial fibrillation. *British Heart Journal* 34, 383–391 (1972).
Reuning, R.H., Sams, R.A. and Notari, R.E., Role of pharmacokinetics in drug dosage adjustment 1: pharmacologic effect kinetics and apparent volume of distribution of digoxin. *Clinical Pharmacology* 13, 127–141 (1973).
Smith, T.W. and Haber, E., Digoxin intoxication: the relationship of clinical presentation to serum digoxin concentration. *Journal of Clinical Investigation* 49, 2377–2386 (1970).

12. BETA-BLOCKING AGENTS

It is generally held that plasma concentrations of β-blockers are related to the effect in any given individual. Nevertheless there is a considerable inter-subject variability in the plasma levels required to produce a certain effect and even more variation in the effective oral dose.

Both the doses necessary to produce effective adrenergic β-blockade and to secure an antihypertensive effect may vary over an extremely wide range, an observation which has been made by many clinicians since the introduction of propranolol as the first efficacious and safe β-blocker in 1966. Such variations have since been described with most other β-blocking agents. The first assays of plasma propranolol levels (Grant et al. 1966) reported in patients with angina pectoris showed huge inter-subject variations, which originally were attributed to differences in absorption. Later research has shown this assumption to be false, since most β-blockers in general use today (except atenolol and oxprenolol) are rapidly and almost completely absorbed. The extreme, sometimes up to twentyfold, variations in plasma propranolol levels have effectively been explained by differences in metabolism (Shand et al. 1970). Drugs like propranolol (Paterson et al. 1970), alprenolol (Åblad et al. 1972) and, to some extent, metoprolol (von Bahr et al. 1976) are exposed to metabolic breakdown by the liver before they can appear in the systemic circulation. The fraction of the absorbed dose which eventually enters the systemic circulation (i.e. the bioavailability) is determined by hepatic extraction, which in turn is a function of hepatic blood flow. Hepatic clearance being high, most of the dose will be eliminated before it can exert any pharmacological effect at the receptor site. The absence of this "first-pass effect" in patients with portocaval anastomosis (Shand and Rangno 1972) is further proof of the importance of this mechanism. Although the apparently complete clearance of low doses of propranolol with the absence of detectable blood levels – see fig. 1 (Shand and Rangno 1971) – has since been attributed to the insensitivity and unspecificity of the plasma assay used (Chidsey et al. 1975; Gomeni et al. 1977) the general principle of the observation is firmly established. If the same dose of the drug is given intravenously, and thus bypasses the hepatic circulation, a much better correlation with the degree of β-blockade is observed (Dollery et al. 1971; Cleaveland and Shand 1972). It will be obvious that such problems do not occur with β-blockers which are metabolized in the liver

to only a minor extent or not at all, e.g. sotalol (Shanks et al. 1975), oxprenolol (Mason and Winer 1976) and atenolol (Shanks et al. 1977). In the case
of metoprolol the issue is less clear; though the difference between the
effects of oral and intravenous doses is slight (Johnsson et al. 1975), and
absorption essentially complete, plasma levels may vary over a 17-fold range
(von Bahr et al. 1976) and there is no correlation between dose and mean
steady-state plasma concentration. The main difficulty still lies in defining
clinical parameters for β-blockade. Criteria which have been used comprise
inhibition of the resting heart rate or of tachycardia during head-up tilting,
inhibition of exercise tachycardia, glycerol trinitrate tachycardia and isoprenaline tachycardia. Though most of these criteria give a fairly close
approximation to the degree of adrenergic β-receptor blockade none of
them is wholly specific or physiological, and none of them has the accuracy
obtained in animal models. By general consensus the inhibition of exercise
tachycardia is considered to be the best test method available, and ꞥ carries
the additional advantage of being a suitable test for the antianginal effects
of these drugs (Alderman and Harrison 1971). The results can be quantified
and they are reproducible from day to day in the same individual (George
et al. 1973).

PHARMACOKINETICS OF BETA-BLOCKERS: CORRELATION OF
CHEMICAL AND PHARMACOLOGICAL KINETICS

The pharmacokinetics of most β-blockers on the market have been extensively studied to the neglect of pharmacodynamic factors. Nevertheless
re-evaluation of the latter has been triggered by pharmacokinetic studies.
Because most β-blockers have relatively short half-lives (table 1) some
manufacturers have introduced longer-acting slow-release forms (alprenolol, oxprenolol and metoprolol); others, after the practolol disaster, have
introduced drugs with long systemic half-lives (atenolol, sotalol) which are
claimed to be suitable for once daily dosage, at least in the treatment of
hypertension. However, such drugs, being less lipid-soluble and more
polar, have the disadvantage of low and often erratic or dose-dependent
bioavailability.
   Surprisingly few studies have been published in which the pharmacological effects in human volunteers and patients have been correlated in time to
the pharmacokinetic behaviour of propranolol. Some patients seem to
behave in a completely different manner from others with the same plasma
levels, both in regard to the degree of β-blockade – see fig. 2 (Zacest and
Koch-Weser 1972) – and to the antihypertensive effect (Weiss et al. 1976).
The bimodal distribution observed in both these investigations suggests
genetic differences in hepatic metabolism. Neither plasma renin activity

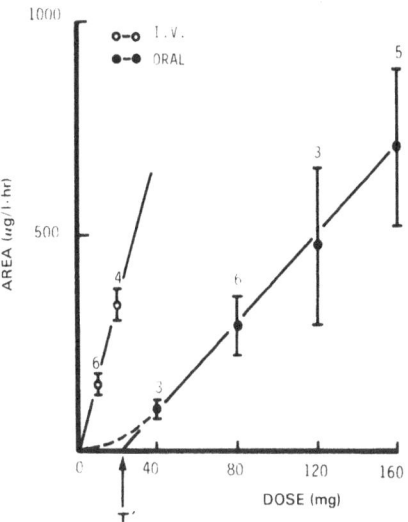

Figure 1. Area under the curve *v* dose of propranolol in six subjects *T* = apparent threshold, i.e. the dose below which no plasma levels are detectable (Shand and Rangno 1971).

Table 1. Pharmacokinetic properties of some β-blockers (Shanks et al. 1975; Johnsson and Regårdh 1976; Mason and Winer 1976).

Drug	Plasma half-life (h)	Apparent volume of distribution (β-phase) (l/kg)	Total drug Clearance (l/min)	Protein binding, (%)	unchanged in urine %	Active metabolites
Propranolol	2–3	3.6	1.0	93	< 1	yes
Alprenolol	2–3	3.0	1.2	85	< 1	yes
Oxprenolol	1.5–2	1.11	0.6	?	?	probably
Pindolol	3–4	2.0	0.4	57	~ 40	no
Metoprolol	3–4	5.6	1.1	12	~ 3	minor fraction
Atenolol	7–9	0.76	0.9	20	> 90	no
Sotalol	7–19	0.78	0.5	?	~ 55	no

nor endogenous adrenergic activity has fully explained such differences. Extremely high propranolol levels have been found in uraemic patients in the absence of the degree of β-blockade expected at such concentrations (Bianchetti et al. 1976). On the other hand, for reasons not yet fully elucidated, plasma levels in patients with acute myocardial infarction remain well below those found in patients with normal myocardial function receiving the same dose (Rutherford et al. 1976). In patients with liver failure the situation is further complicated since hepatic elimination decreases, the volume of distribution, particularly in patients with ascites, increases, and diminished protein binding causes an increase in the fraction

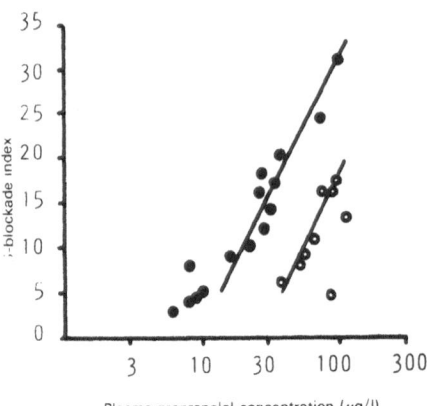

Figure 2. Relationship of plasma propranolol concentration to degree of β-blockade in 23 patients. Open and closed circles identify two distinct groups (Zacest and Koch-Weser 1972).

of unbound, pharmacologically active, drug in the plasma (Branch et al. 1976).

However, in the great majority of patients plasma concentrations and adrenergic β-receptor blocking effect correlate quite well. Preliminary studies by Cleaveland and Shand (1972) had shown a linear correlation between the logarithm of plasma propranolol levels over a range of 25–150 μg/l and the effect, quantitatively expressed as "dose ratio," DR (i.e., the ratio of the CD_{25}, the chronotropic dose of isoprenaline required to raise the resting heart rate by 25 beats per minute, after propranolol to the CD_{25} before administration of the drug), both after oral and intravenous administration. This parameter seemed to correlate quite well with the degree of inhibition of exercise tachycardia (McDevitt and Shand 1975). The effect, expressed as DR–1, declined linearly in time with a pharmacological half-life only slightly exceeding the half-life of the plasma concentration of the intravenously administered drug. It has been suggested (McDevitt et al. 1976) that the plasma level of unbound propranolol (approximated by the assay of red cell concentrations) correlated even better with DR–1. However, during chronic oral treatment important differences came to light; the half-life increases as treatment continues, probably both through saturation of hepatic binding and a reduction in hepatic extraction (Evans and Shand 1973a, Chidsey et al. 1975); despite the short systemic half-life, accumulation occurs and the fraction of the drug in the blood not bound to red cells increases (Evans and Shand 1973b), i.e., the pharmacological effects of the drug delay its own elimination (Nies et al. 1973). The importance of haemodynamic factors has been clearly demonstrated by Weiss et al. (1976); cardiac output closely correlates with both propranolol half-

life ($r = 0.72$) and total drug clearance ($r = 0.96$) in man. Similar results
have been reported with other β-blockers.

DISSOCIATION OF EFFECT AND PLASMA CONCENTRATION

Paterson et al. (1970) found that in some subjects the pharmacological
half-life of propranolol as assessed by the increase in the dose of isoprenaline required to raise the heart rate by 20 beats per minute considerably
exceeded plasma half-life (fig. 3). Similar observations have been made with
alprenolol (Åblad et al. 1972) and pindolol (Olsson and Varnauskas 1973)
using inhibition of exercise tachycardia and isoprenaline antagonism
respectively as parameters of β-blockade. Up to 14 percent inhibition of
exercise tachycardia can still be demonstrated seven hours after the
administration of 200 mg alprenolol at plasma concentrations below 10
μg/l. The interpretation of such conflicting results is further complicated
by the apparent lack of agreement on the duration of the effect as measured
by these two methods: Achong et al. (1976) reported that whereas inhibition
of exercise tachycardia after a single intravenous dose of propranolol or
timolol had disappeared after nine hours, the response to isoprenaline was
still partly (but statistically significantly) blocked 24 hours after administration of these drugs. This observation fits in with the results of the experiments reported by Faulkner et al. (1973): left atrial tissue removed during

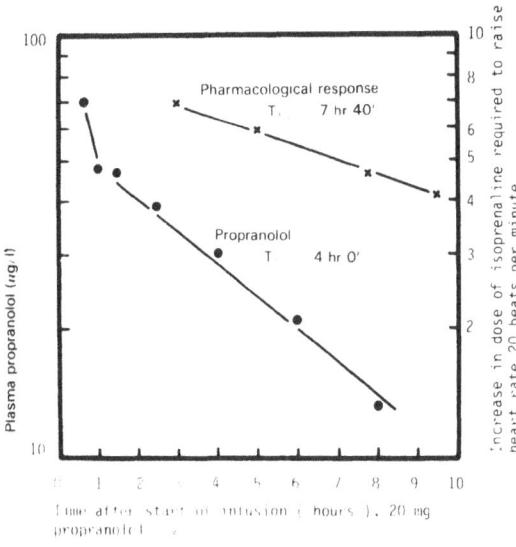

Figure 3. Difference between pharmacological and chemical half-life, $T_{1/2}$, of propranolol
(Paterson et al. 1970).

cardiac surgery 48 hours after withdrawal of chronic propranolol therapy may still show up to 40 percent blockade of the *in vitro* response to iso-prenaline, though with the available methods no trace of propranolol is detectable in such tissues. Others (Kanto et al. 1976; Brundin et al. 1976) have confirmed these observations: 24 hours after the oral administration of propranolol, though plasma levels have fallen below the limit of detection, negative chronotropic and inotropic effects of the drug are still easily demonstrable, both in volunteers and hypertensive subjects. Investigations set up to determine whether such discrepancies may be explained by the formation of pharmacologically active metabolites (i.e. 4-hydroxy-pro-pranolol and 4-hydroxy-alprenolol) have been remarkably unsuccessful; the half-life of such metabolites is generally extremely short, and their role in chronic treatment seems restricted (Dollery et al. 1971; Åblad et al. 1974).

DOSE-EFFECT RELATIONSHIP IN THE TREATMENT OF HYPERTENSION

Though the clinical effect, the absolute or relative decrease in blood pres-sure, can be quantitatively assessed without great difficulty, the mechanism of action of β-blockers in hypertension is far from clear, and this complicates the interpretation of plasma levels in patients receiving such treatment. The inhibition of plasma renin activity seems to have been ruled out as a decisive factor; central mechanisms may only be operative in patients treated with β-blockers which pass the blood-brain barrier, and cardiac β-blockade obviously does not explain the whole effect. Beta-blockade is essentially complete at relatively low propranolol levels: Chidsey et al. (1976) determined a "threshold" level of 100 μg/l, achieved at a dose of approximately 80 mg t.i.d., but further increases of dose will cause signifi-cant progressive decreases in blood pressure (Amery 1975; Lehtonen et al. 1977; Zweifler and Esler 1977). Similar observations have been made with atenolol (Amery et al. 1977), metoprolol (Brogden et al. 1977) and pindolol (Anavekar et al. 1975; Weiss et al. 1977). In general, the pharmacological half-life of the hypotensive effect is approximately two to four times as long as the systemic half-life. Whereas pindolol and propranolol (half-lives 2–4 h) have a fairly long duration of antihypertensive action, sometimes lasting up to 24 hours after the last dose (Wilson et al. 1976), the hypotensive effect of a β-blocker with a very short half-life, such as oxprenolol, does not exceed 8 h (Mason and Winer 1976), though the drug does provide smooth blood pressure control over 24 hours if given in divided doses (Materson et al. 1976). On the other hand the effect of drugs with long systemic half-lives like atenolol (McAinsh 1977) or sotalol (Shanks et al. 1975) may last up to 48 hours after the administration of a single oral dose. During chronic treatment the relationship between dose and effect often disappears completely, blood pressure showing a gradual further fall in time though dose remains constant. Brundin et al. (1976) concluded that long-term β-blockade leads to a physiological adaptation of haemodynamic mechanisms (Resetting of baroceptors?) since patients who had been treated with propranolol for two to nine months were completely unresponsive to the acute administration of a single intravenous dose of the drug given three days after withdrawal of the oral treatment. Disappointingly few critical investigations on the relationship between plasma levels and the antihypertensive response to adrenergic β-blockade have been published. Whereas Lehtonen et al. (1977) found no correlation with plasma propranolol levels at all, Esler et al. (1977) postulated a dual mechanism: some patients with increased catecholamine secretion and high plasma renin activity showed substantial falls in blood pressure at low plasma propranolol levels – the relation to plasma concentration being indistinct and non-predictable – whereas others only responded at high levels, and this response was in no way related to plasma renin activity or catecholamine secretion. A similar dual mechanism had already been proposed by Shand et al. (1975), who speculated that the response at higher levels was in some way related to a central hypotensive effect. However, this hypothesis cannot explain similar antihypertensive effects caused by atenolol, which does not cross the blood-brain barrier to any appreciable extent. Mean steady-state plasma concentrations of metoprolol (von Bahr et al. 1976) did not correlate with the antihypertensive effect at all, though they did show a relationship with the degree of β-blockade. Thus far only pindolol plasma levels appear to correlate in any way with the antihypertensive response (Weiss et al. 1977).

UNDER WHAT CONDITIONS DOES THE HYPOTENSIVE RESPONSE TO PROPRANOLOL FOLLOW PHARMACOLOGICAL RULES?

We (Krediet, Offerhaus and Dunning, 1979) investigated the relationship of plasma propranolol levels and the hypotensive response in 16 patients with severe uncomplicated essential hypertension. Plasma propranolol was assayed using an improved fluorometric method (Offerhaus and van der Vecht 1976). Mean steady-state propranolol levels (C_{ss}) were calculated from the area under the curve during a 12-hour interval at a dosage of 80 mg b.i.d. using the trapezoid rule (Collste et al. 1976a, 1976b). Though a statistically significant ($p < 0.005$) correlation was demonstrated between the proportional decrease in mean arterial pressure and the inhibition of exercise tachycardia (proving the importance of β-blockade as the main hypotensive mechanism) there was no correlation at all between the hypotensive effect (measured as the proportional fall of systolic, diastolic and

mean arterial pressure) and mean steady-state plasma propranolol concentration. We could therefore in no way confirm the close correlation
between these parameters at propranolol levels below 100 µg/l as reported
by Zweifler and Esler (1977). However, there is a fairly strong indication
that the logarithm of the mean steady-state plasma level over a certain
"threshold" value of approximately 50 µg/l correlates with the final blood
pressure level obtained after six weeks treatment (fig. 4). The same correlation was found when instead of the complicated calculation of C_{ss} one
employed the plasma level, C_{12}, just before the next dose (fig. 5). However,
blood pressure response at low mean steady-state levels (< 50 µg/l, $C_{12} <$
10 µg/l) seems to be independent of plasma concentration. This finding fits
in with the "dual mechanism" concept as postulated by Shand et al. (1975)
and Esler et al. (1977), though our results must lead to the conclusion that
β-blockade is the predominant hypotensive mechanism operative at high
plasma propranolol concentrations. The number of studies which we have
so far performed with higher doses (160 mg b.i.d.) is too limited to permit any
conclusions. In addition our observations confirmed the existence of
similarly wide variations in plasma level after a single fixed oral dose as
reported by Zacest and Koch-Weser (1972), Evans and Shand (1973a) and
Chidsey et al. (1975), though these variations tend to be less during chronic
treatment (fig. 6).

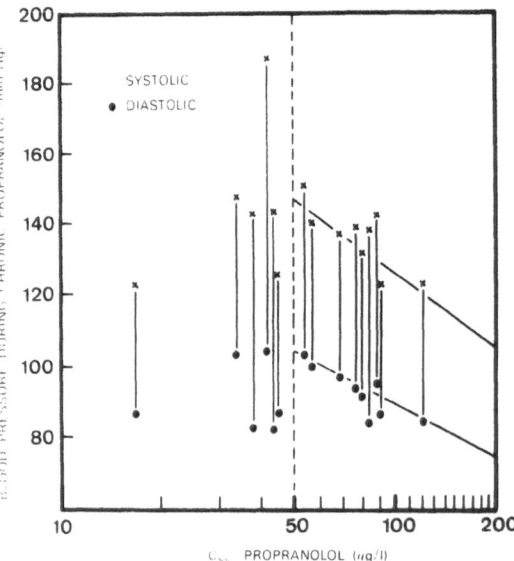

Figure 4. Relationship of steady-state propranolol concentration and systolic and diastolic
blood pressure levels obtained after chronic treatment of 15 hypertensive patients with
80 mg b.i.d.

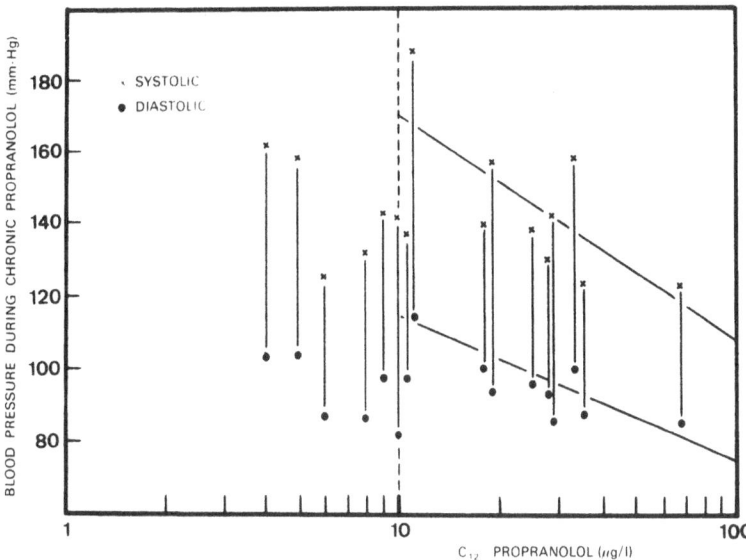

Figure 5. Relationship of plasma propranolol concentration, assayed at the end of the dosing interval (C_{12}) and systolic and diastolic blood pressure levels obtained after chronic treatment of 16 hypertensive patients with 80 mg b.i.d.

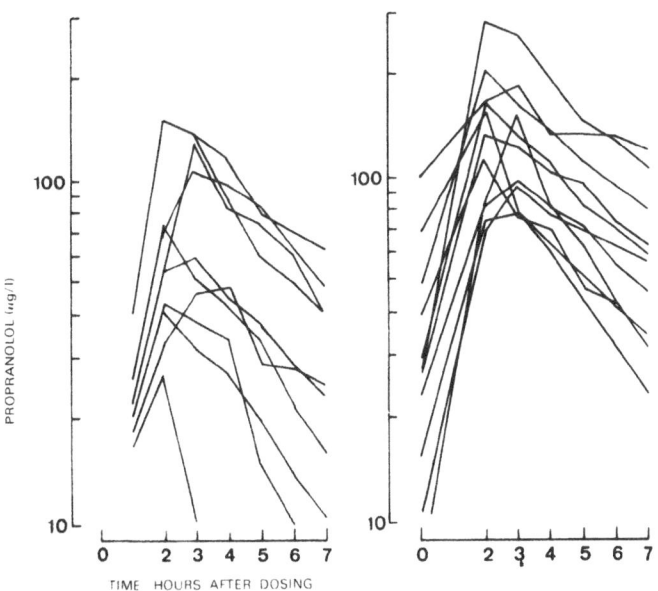

Figure 6. Individual plasma propranolol concentration *v* time curves in 11 hypertensive patients after a single dose of 80 mg between (left) and after (right) chronic treatment with 80 mg b.i.d.

RECOMMENDATIONS CONCERNING THE RATIONALE OF AND
INDICATIONS FOR PLASMA LEVEL ASSAYS OF BETA-BLOCKERS

If plasma levels of β-blockers are determined at all the following principles
may be used as guidelines:

1. With the exception of propranolol, a substance which because of its
chemical structure can without great difficulty be assayed with a satisfactory
degree of sensitivity and specificity using fluorometric methods, the chemical assay of β-blockers in plasma is difficult and time-consuming, involving
extraction, formation of a fluorinated derivative and quantitative determination by gas-liquid chromatography using the often capricious and
laborious method of electron capture detection (Walle 1974). All solvents
used should be absolutely halogen-free (so-called "Pesticide Grade"), and
these are therefore difficult to obtain and expensive.

2. Randomly timed assays, except when they are required to check
patient compliance, should never be performed in view of the wide variations in plasma level and marked inter-subject variations. Careful timing is
therefore essential; plasma samples should be collected after establishment
of the elimination phase of the drug, e.g. at least four to five hours after the
last dose. Samples taken at a later point in time may yield very low values,
which are difficult to measure and to interpret. Because the area under the
curve correlates with the amount of drug available in the body, and, at

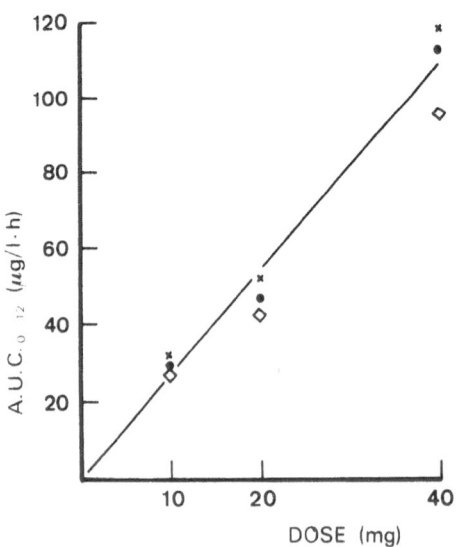

Figure 7. Relationship between area values and low doses of propranolol in three patients
(Gomeni et al. 1977).

least at low doses, (fig. 7) with oral dose, calculation of the mean steady-state concentration is still the best method available, but it necessitates the collection of six or seven carefully timed samples. Peak concentrations (C_{max}) do also correlate with C_{ss}, but the variability over 150 $\mu g/l$ is high and there is a wide variation in the time at which C_{max} is reached (figs. 6 and 8).

3. The assay of plasma levels should be limited to patients with dysrhythmias and angina pectoris, in whom the therapeutic effect more or less (depending on the degree of metabolism of the drug in question) correlates with the plasma concentration. In such patients it has been repeatedly shown that the plasma concentration of most β-blockers is fairly closely correlated to the degree of adrenergic β-blockade. Even these data obtained in one patient are not automatically valid for any other patient because of wide inter-subject variations in plasma level and the absence of any correlation with dose (or at least with high doses) even with drugs which are hardly or not at all metabolized.

The rationale of performing such assays is most evident when one is

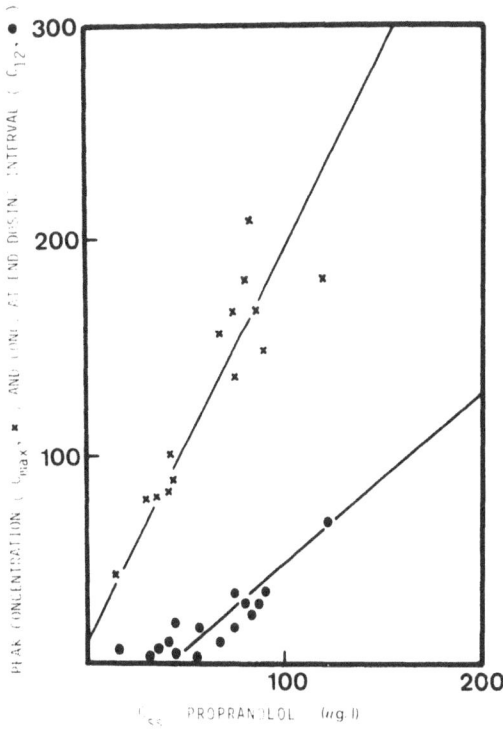

Figure 8. Correlation between steady-state plasma concentration (C_{ss}) peak concentration (C_{max}) and the concentration at the end of the dosing interval (C_{12}) during chronic treatment of hypertensive patients with propranolol, 80 mg b.i.d.

dealing with drugs with a high hepatic extraction rate (propranolol and alprenolol) and with drugs having low and dose-dependent or erratic bio-availability (sotalol, atenolol, metoprolol and oxprenolol). Obviously plasma-level assays will provide only scant information if the profile of the dose-response curve is comparatively flat, as in the use of atenolol for the treatment of hypertension. Only with pindolol is the dose itself likely to be a far simpler and better guide.

4. Plasma concentration studies in hypertensive patients treated with β-blockers have shown that adrenergic β-blockade as such, which is essentially complete at relatively low plasma levels, does not fully explain the hypotensive properties of this class of drug, because the hypotensive effect seems to remain dose-dependent at plasma levels far exceeding those needed for full β-blockade. Evidence, however, is still conflicting, and the issue is far from solved. Particularly at low plasma levels other mechanisms, i.e. increased concentrations at receptor sites other than those involved in myocardial β-blockade (Renin suppression?) may be operative.

Accordingly, the assay of plasma levels of β-blockers in the treatment of hypertension in clinical practice has no rationale except as a research tool, but it might be useful in the detection of non-compliance, a surprisingly common shortcoming in any therapeutic situation.

REFERENCES

Åblad, B., Borg, K.O. and Johnsson, G. Life Sci. 14, 693–704 (1974).
Åblad, B., Ervik, M., Hallgren, J., Johnsson, G. and Sölvell, L., Europ. J. Clin. Pharmacol. 5, 44–52 (1972).
Achong, M.R., Piafsky, K.M. and Ogilvie, R.I., Clin. Pharmacol. Therap. 19, 148–153 (1976).
Alderman, E.L. and Harrison, D.C., In: Circulatory Effects and Clinical Uses of Beta-Adrenergic Blocking Drugs. Ed., Harrison, D.C., Amsterdam, 1971.
Amery, A., In: Pathophysiology and Management of Arterial Hypertension. Ed., Berglund, G., Hansson, L. and Werkö, L., Gothenburg, 1975.
Amery, A., Lijnen. P., Fagard, R. and Reijbrouck, T., Postgrad. Med. J. 53, Suppl. 3, 116–120 (1977).
Anavekar, S.N., Louis, W.J., Morgan, T.O., Doyle, A.E. and Johnston, C.I., Clin. Exp. Pharmacol. Physiol. 2, 203–212 (1975).
Von Bahr, C., Collste, P., Frisk-Holmberg, M., Haglund, K., Jorfelt, L., Orme, M.L'E., Östman, J. and Sjøqvist, F., Clin. Pharmacol. Therap. 20, 130–137 (1976).
Bianchetti, G., Graziani, G., Brancaccio, D., Morganti, A., Leonetti, G., Manfrin, N., Sega, R., Gomeni. R., Ponticelli, C. and Morselli, P.L., Clin. Pharmacokin. 1, 373–384 (1976).
Branch, R.A., James, J. and Read. A.E., Brit. J. Clin. Pharmacol. 3, 324–328 (1976).
Brogden, R.N., Heel, R.C., Speight, T.M. and Avery, G.S., Drugs 14, 321–348 (1977).
Brundin, T., Edhag, O. and Lundman, T., Brit. Heart J. 38, 1065–1072 (1976).
Chidsey, C.A., Morselli, P., Bianchetti, G., Morganti, A., Leonetti, G. and Zanchetti, A., Circulation 52, 313–318 (1975).
Chidsey, C.A., Pine. M., Favrot, L., Smith, S., Leonetti, G., Morselli, P. and Zanchetti, A., Postgrad. Med. J. 52, Suppl. 4, 26–32 (1977).
Cleaveland, C.R. and Shand, D.G., Clin. Pharmacol. Therap. 13, 181–185 (1972).

Collste, P., Haglund, K., Frisk-Holmberg, M., Orme, M.L'E., Rawlins, M.D. and Östman, J., *Europ. J. Clin. Pharmacol.* 10, 89–96 (1976a).
Collste, P., Haglund, K., Frisk-Homberg, M. and Rawlins, M.D., *Europ. J. Clin Pharmacol.* 10, 85–88 (1976b).
Dollery, C.T., Davies, D.S. and Connolly, M.E., *Ann. N.Y. Acad. Sci.* 179, 108–114 (1971).
Esler, M., Zweifler, A., Randall, O. and Dequattro, V., *Clin. Pharmacol. Therap.* 22, 299–308 (1977).
Evans, G.H. and Shand, D.G., *Clin. Pharmacol. Therap.* 14, 487–493 (1973a).
Evans, G.H. and Shand, D.G., *Clin. Pharmacol. Therap.* 14, 494–500 (1973b).
Faulkner, S.L., Hopkins, J.T., Boerth, R.C., Young, J.L., Nies, A.S., Bender, H.W. and Shand, D.G., *New Engl. J. Med.* 289, 607–609 (1973).
George, C.F., Fenyvesi, T. and Dollery, C.T. In: *Biological Effects of Drugs in Relation to Their Plasma Concentrations.* Ed., Davies, D.S. and Prichard, B.N.C., London, 1973.
Gomeni, R., Bianchetti, G., Sega, R. and Morselli, P.L., *J. Pharmacokin. Biopharm.* 5, 183–192 (1977).
Grant, R.H.E., Keelan, P., Kernohan, R.J., Leonard, J.C., Nancekievill, L. and Sinclair, K., *Amer. J. Cardiol.* 18, 361–365 (1966).
Johnsson, G. and Regårdh, C.-G., *Clin. Pharmacokin.* 1, 233–263 (1976).
Johnsson, G., Regårdh, C.-G. and Sölvell, L., *Acta Pharmacol. Toxicol.* 36, Suppl. 5, 31–44 (1975).
Kanto, J., Kleimola, T., Mäntylä, R. and Syvälahti, E., *Acta Pharmacol. Toxicol.* 39, 573–576 (1976).
Lehtonen, A., Kanto, J. and Kleimola, T., *Europ. J. Clin. Pharmacol.* 11, 155–160 (1977).
McAinsh, J., *Postgrad. Med. J.* 53, Suppl. 3, 74–78 (1977).
McDevitt, D.G. and Shand, D.G., *Clin. Pharmacol. Therap.* 18, 708–713 (1975).
McDevitt, D.G., Frisk-Holmberg, M., Hollifield, J.W. and Shand, D.G., *Clin. Pharmacol. Therap.* 20, 152–157 (1976).
Mason, W.D. and Winer, N., *Clin. Pharmacol. Therap.* 20, 401–412 (1976).
Materson, B.J., Michael, U.F., Oster, J.R., Perez-Stable, E.C., Hernandez, A. and Smith, M., *Clin. Pharmacol. Therap.* 20, 142–151 (1976).
Nies, A.S., Evans, G.H. and Shand, D.G., *J. Pharmacol. Expt. Therap.* 184, 716–720 (1973).
Offerhaus, L. and van der Vecht, J., *Brit. J. Clin. Pharmacol.* 3, 1061–1062 (1976).
Olsson, S.B. and Varnauskas, E., *Europ. J. Clin. Pharmacol.* 5, 214–217 (1973).
Paterson, J.W., Connolly, M.E., Dollery, C.T., Hayes, A. and Cooper, R.G., *Pharmacol. Clin.* 2, 127–133 (1970).
Rutherford, J.D., Singh, B.N., Ambler, P.K. and Morris, R.M., *Clin. Exp. Pharmacol. Physiol.* 3, 297–304 (1976).
Shand, D.G. and Rangno, R.E., *Pharmacology* 7, 159–168 (1971).
Shand, D.G., Frisk-Holmberg, M., McDevitt D.G., Sherman, K. and Hollifield, J. In: *Pathophysiology and Management of Arterial Hypertension.* Ed., Berglund, G., Hansson, L. and Werkö, L., Gothenburg, 1975.
Shand, D.G., Nuckolls, E.M. and Oates, J.A., *Clin. Pharmacol. Therap.* 11, 112–120 (1970).
Shanks, R.G., Brown, H.C., Carruthers, S.G. and Kelly, J.G., In: *Advances in Beta-Adrenergic Blocking Therapy.* Ed., Snart, A.G. *Sotalol.* Amsterdam (1975).
Shanks, R.G., Carruthers, S.G., Kelly, J.G. and McDevitt, D.G., *Postgrad. Med. J.* 53, Suppl. 3, 70–73 (1977).
Walle, T., *J. Pharm. Sci.* 63, 1885–1891 (1974).
Weiss, Y.A., Loria, Y., Safar, M.E., Lavene, D.E., Simon, A.C., Georges, D.R. and Milliez, P.L., *Curr. Therap. Res.* 21, 644–655 (1977).
Weiss, Y.A., Safar, M.E., Chevillard, C., Frydman, A., Simon, A., Lemaire, P. and Alexandre, J.M., *Europ. J. Clin. Pharmacol.* 10, 387–392 (1976).
Wilson, M., Morgan, G. and Morgan, T. *Brit. J. Clin. Pharmacol.* 3, 857–861 (1976).
Zacest, R. and Koch-Weser, J., *Pharmacology* 7, 178–184 (1972).
Zweifler, A. and Esler, M., *Amer. J. Cardiol.* 40, 105–109 (1977).

13. PROCAINAMIDE AND QUINIDINE

F.A. DE WOLFF

Procainamide (PA) and Quinidine (QD) have a number of pharmacological and therapeutic properties in common, which justifies the discussion of these two drugs together in one chapter. Both are effective antiarrhythmic drugs which exert their action on the heart by delaying the repolarization of myocardial cells and increasing the refractory period. Both drugs are often regarded in therapeutics as interchangeable, but PA may be less effective than QD in atrial arrhythmias and more effective in ventricular arrhythmias. PA and QD both have a small therapeutic index. Their clinical application is complicated by the fact that symptoms of overdosage often resemble those of the disease itself. In addition, even at low doses and serum concentrations, allergic side effects are not uncommon. These effects may present for example as systemic lupus erythematosus (SLE) with PA and immune thrombocytopenia with QD. Like their pharmacodynamic actions, the pharmacokinetic properties of PA and QD are much alike, which is surprising, since the chemical structures of the two drugs differ greatly (figs. 1 and 2).

Both are basic drugs with a plasma half-life of approximately four hours, but that for QD is sometimes longer. The apparent volume of distribution is approximately 2 l/kg. QD is 70–80 percent plasma protein bound, whereas

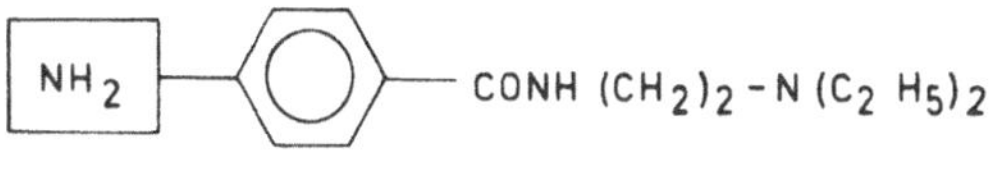

Procainamide

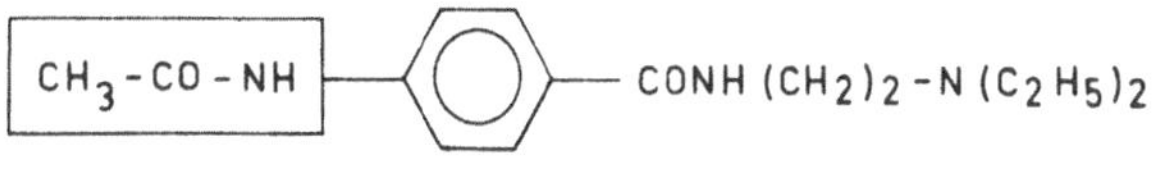

N – acetylprocainamide
(NAPA)

Figure 1. Structures of procainamide (PA) and its N-acetylated metabolite (NAPA).

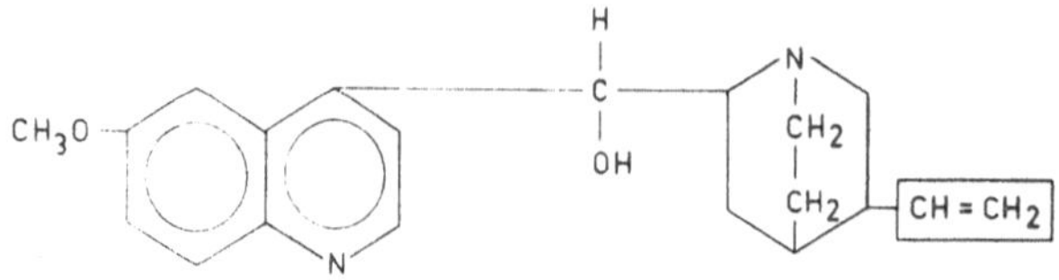

Quinidine

Dihydroquinidine : $-CH_2-CH_3$

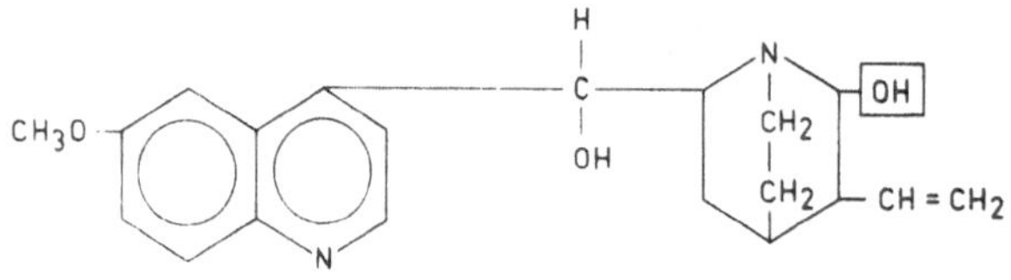

Quinidine metabolite I

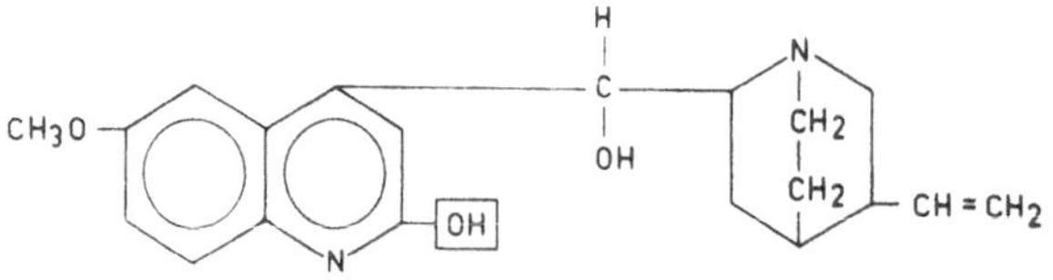

Quinidine metabolite II

Figure 2. Structures of quinidine (QD), dihydroquinidine (DHQD) and two hydroxylated metabolites of QD (Conn and Luchi 1964).

PA is only 15 percent bound. The most notable difference between PA and QD is the way in which the drugs are metabolized. Since consideration of their metabolism is of utmost importance for the interpretation of the serum concentrations of the drugs, these metabolic aspects will be discussed separately.

WHY DETERMINE SERUM LEVELS?

In clinical practice, careful thought is usually given to choosing an appropriate drug for a patient, but relatively little attention is paid to establishing the most effective dosage schedule. It is, however, not a drug *per se* which has a certain effect, but rather a given concentration of that drug at its site of action (Koch-Weser 1977). Although serum levels do not necessarily reflect the actual concentration of a drug at its receptor, these serum concentrations are generally considered to be a good working index for the situation at the site of action. Antiarrhythmics form a good practical example of a group of drugs whereby at some serum levels no action is perceived, whereas at other, higher levels, toxic effects are observed. Between these extremes lies a range of concentrations which are consistent with optimal therapeutic results and are characteristic for each drug. In the treatment of cardiac arrhythmias, the prescribing of so-called "average" or "usual" doses of antiarrhythmic drugs is still common practice. This often leads to therapeutic failures or to serious toxic effects. An explanation for this phenomenon has been given for PA by Koch-Weser (1977). Steady-state PA levels were determined in a group of 325 inpatients under various PA regimes. From fig. 3 it is obvious that there is no positive correlation whatsoever between dosage and serum level. In other words, in different

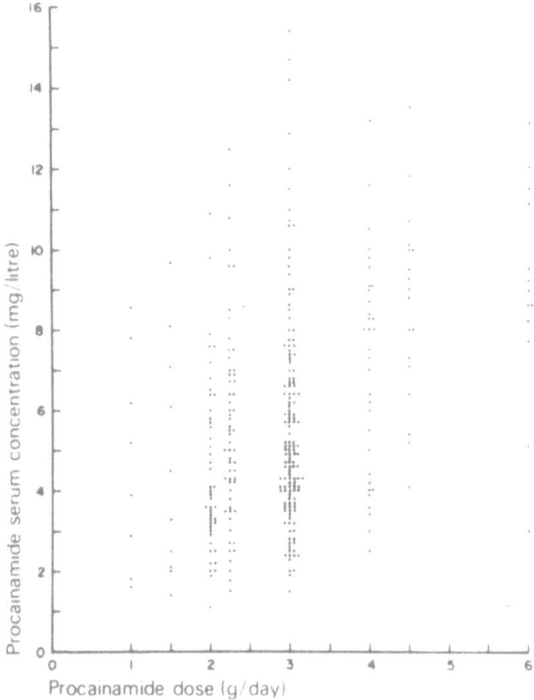

Figure 3. Serum concentrations of procainamide in 325 hospitalized patients receiving 0.25, 0.375 or 0.5 g of the hydrochloride orally every 6, 4 or 3 hours. Serum levels represent averages of at least two values after achievement of steady state (after Koch-Weser: Clinical Pharmacokinetics 2:389, 1977; by permission of author and editor).

patients a given dose of PA yields widely different serum concentrations of the drug. From analysis of these data and clinical observations (fig. 4) it was found that in most patients a serum concentration below 4 mg/l was ineffective in the treatment of ventricular arrhythmias. About 90 percent of the patients responded well to a concentration between 4 and 8 mg/l. In this range, serious cardiovascular toxicity was never observed. Arrhythmias in an additional 10 percent of patients who did not respond were controlled by serum concentrations between 8 and 12 mg/l. However, at these levels serious toxicity, such as dysrhythmias, was also observed. Concentrations above 12 mg/l were almost never effective where lower serum levels had not achieved a response. A concentration above 16 mg/l PA can be lethal. Exceptions to these statements are rare, but they nevertheless exist. Recently a patient was admitted to our hospital with ventricular tachycardia after a severe myocardial infarction. The tachycardia was refractory to any drug except PA in very high dosage (15 g/day intravenously). The serum levels of PA were around 25 mg/l, but as soon as the serum levels dropped below 20 mg/l the tachycardia reappeared. No toxic symptoms were perceived (de Wolff et al., to be published).

From the studies of Koch-Weser it can be concluded that, at least for PA, the serum concentration has, in general, to be kept in a certain range to achieve an optimal antiarrhythmic effect. Unfortunately, a comparable extensive study on QD has never been described, although many thousands of pages have been written about this alkaloid since the first reports of its efficacy (Frey 1918a, 1918b). However, from a combination of data it can be shown that there is also a therapeutic range for QD. It is, however, not easy to determine what this range actually is, since at least eight different "therapeutic ranges" have been proposed (table 1). This discrepancy can be attributed to the fact that there is no agreement about "what" and "how

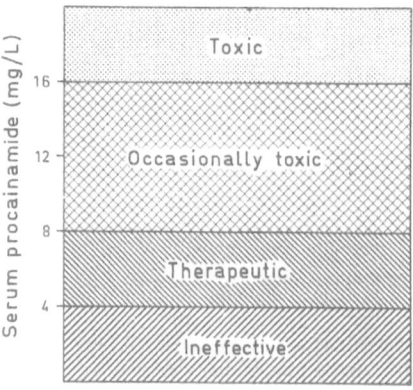

Figure 4. Relationship between serum concentrations of procainamide and clinical response.

Table 1. Proposed therapeutic ranges for quinidine.

Serum concentration (mg/l)	Method type[a]	Reference
1–4	B	Gey et al. (1975)
1–5	C	Moulin and Kinsun (1977)
2–4	?	Sjöqvist et al. (1976)
2–5	B	Soeterboek and van Thiel (1976)
2.3–5.0	B	Kessler et al. (1974)
3–6	?	Sloman (1976)
4–8	A	Elevitch (1973)
4–9	B	Kutsch Lojenga (1972)

a. Type A: measuring total amount of cinchona alkaloids;
Type B: measuring unmetabolized quinidine and dihydroquinidine;
Type C: measuring only unmetabolized quinidine.

what" should be measured in QD therapy. The specificity of the analytical method determines, among other things, the concentration range considered as therapeutic. Thus for instance, it is important whether metabolites should be co-assayed or not.

CHOICE OF ASSAY METHOD WITH RESPECT TO METABOLISM

Procainamide

Attention is therefore now focused upon the question which method should be chosen for both PA and QD, with respect to their metabolic pattern. Since PA is the better investigated of the two drugs, its metabolism first will be considered in relation to its effect. The most important metabolite of PA is N-acetylprocainamide, or NAPA (see fig. 1). In the last four years it has been demonstrated that NAPA has antiarrhythmic activity (Drayer et al. 1974; Refsum et al. 1975). NAPA is formed from PA by the action of the liver enzyme N-acetyltransferase (Gibson, Matusik et al. 1975; Frislid et al. 1976; Lunde et al. 1977; Karlsson 1978). The activity of this enzyme is genetically determined. All drugs that are metabolized in this way are subject to a bimodal acetylation in man. The population ratio of rapid versus slow acetylators varies widely between ethnic groups throughout the world: in people of eastern Asian origin more than 90 percent are rapid acetylators, whereas of Egyptians only 20 percent are rapid metabolizers and 30–40 percent of Western Europeans acetylate rapidly. Fast metabolizers have a much higher NAPA to PA ratio in serum than slow acetylators. This ratio may vary between 0.6 and 5 (Frislid et al. 1975). This means that at a given PA concentration in serum, say 5 mg/l, the NAPA concentration in one patient may be 3 mg/l, but in another patient 25 mg/l. At 5 mg/l PA the sum total of the drug plus the active metabolite may there-

fore be in the range of 8 to 30 mg/l. From these data it might appear that for
therapeutic monitoring both PA and NAPA should be determined. There
are, however, two reasons why this should not be unconditionally accepted.
In the first place, the earlier work of Koch-Weser and Klein (1971) on the
establishment of the therapeutic range was based upon an assay method
which is specific for the unchanged drug. Secondly, to this day it remains
unclear how important the therapeutic effects of NAPA are in patients treated
with PA. The two compounds have different, and at times even opposing,
electrophysiological effects on heart muscle. It is therefore probable that
the potency ratios of PA and NAPA are different for various disturbances
(Koch-Weser 1977). When NAPA was found to have antiarrhythmic properties, it seemed necessary to measure the sum total of PA and NAPA for
therapeutic monitoring. This is done, for instance, after *in vitro* acid hydrolysis of NAPA to PA. Such an assay method is not advocated, since there is
considerable uncertainty about the relative potencies of the drug and the
metabolite. Therefore, the following conclusion can be drawn: for daily
clinical practice, a simple colourimetric (Koch-Weser and Klein 1971;
Sitar et al. 1976), fluorometric (Sterling et al. 1974; Ambler and Masarei
1976) or gas chromatographic (Atkinson et al. 1972) procedure specific for
PA will do. However, if there are unexpected phenomena even in the
therapeutic range, NAPA concentrations may give additional information,
such as in impairment of renal function. For the assay of PA and NAPA in
one procedure, several methods have been described, using gas chromatography (Frislid et al. 1975), high-performance liquid chromatography
(Carr et al. 1976; Dutcher and Strong 1977; Rocco et al. 1977; Shukur et al.
1977; Weddle and Mason 1977) and thin-layer densitometry (Wesley-
Hadzija and Mattocks 1977). As yet no comparative study has been performed to establish which one of these method gives the best result. When
starting up a PA monitoring service and having one of these chromatographic instruments at one's disposal, is it perhaps worthwhile to start with
a procedure giving NAPA concentrations in addition to PA levels. However,
one should be well aware that both concentrations cannot simply be sum-
mated. Extensive clinical studies on patients with various arrhythmias are
required to establish the value of NAPA concentrations.

Phenotyping of the acetylator status
Knowledge of the acetylator phenotype of the actual patient may give a
better chance of optimalizing PA treatment. This knowledge is also of
prognostic value: for instance, slow acetylators have a higher incidence
of immunological side effects than fast acetylators. Phenotyping is a rather
simple procedure: it can be performed by giving the patient a single dose of a
sulfonamide, usually 500 mg sulfadimidine (Evans 1969), and measuring the
metabolite to total drug ratio in urine by the classical colourimetric method

of Bratton and Marshall (1939). With chromatographic techniques pheno-typing can also be done simply by determining the NAPA to total amide ratio in serum or urine (Karlsson 1978). However, the NAPA to PA ratio is not only determined by the acetylator status, since impairment of renal function may also influence this. Both PA and NAPA are excreted by the kidney. In patients with a normal renal function, the elimination of NAPA is slower than that of PA, but in patients with impaired renal function NAPA may even accumulate in the blood (Gibson, Lowenthal et al. 1975; Galeazzi, Sheiner et al. 1976; Drayer et al. 1977; Lima and Jusko 1978). Plasma half-life of NAPA in these patients may be several days instead of the usual several hours. This implies that the NAPA to PA ratio may not only be high in rapid metabolizers, but also in slow metabolizers with impaired renal function. One patient with renal failure has been described in whose plasma NAPA was detectable 38 days after PA was stopped (Drayer et al. 1977). This indicates that in patients with impaired renal function, the concentrations of both PA and NAPA should be determined.

Quinidine

As mentioned before, there is much disagreement about the concentration range of QD that should be considered as "therapeutic" (table 1). Un-fortunately, no extensive clinical studies with QD like that of Koch-Weser for PA have been published. This is in spite of the profusion of assay methods that have been described. These procedures can be divided into three groups. Type A comprises procedures in which all cinchona alka-loids present in serum are assayed (Brodie and Udenfriend 1943; Hamfelt and Malers 1963; Osinga and de Wolff 1976). With Type B methods both QD and dihydroquinidine are determined (Cramér and Isaksson 1963; Armand and Badinand 1972; Kutsch Lojenga 1972; Mulder and Faber 1973; Valentine et al. 1976; Crouthamel et al. 1977; Powers and Sadee 1978). In the third group of methods, Type C, only QD and no other cin-chona alkaloids are determined, or discrimination of QD and dihydroquini-dine was not described (Midha and Charette 1974; Steyn and Hundt 1975; Christiansen 1976; Moulin and Kinsun 1977). Several studies have been performed for the analysis of the difference between the several methods (Härtel and Harjanne 1969; Huffman and Hignite 1976; Osinga and de Wolff 1976).

Before these procedures can be evaluated and a therapeutic range tenta-tively established, the metabolism and the activity of QD and its derivatives have to be discussed. Pharmaceutical preparations of QD are never pure. They all contain a variable amount of dihydroquinidine (DHQD), ranging from 3 to 22 percent (Soeterboek and van Thiel 1976). This compound only differs from QD in that the vinyl side chain is saturated (see fig. 2). Dihydro-quinidine, which is in its pure form also available as a drug, has the same antiarrhythmic effects as QD, and is perhaps even more potent (Scott et al. 1945). It should be noted that DHQD is *not* a metabolite of QD in man. QD itself is metabolized by hydroxylation into at least two major metabolites (see fig. 2). The first has probably no antiarrhythmic potency; the second has been shown to possess antiarrhythmic effects *in vitro* (Conn and Luchi 1964). Clinical experiments to test the effectiveness of the metabolites in man have never been described. It will now be clear that it is so far *un*clear which method should be used for therapeutic monitoring of QD. It is recommended that DHQD should always be co-assayed, since it is a potent drug which is present in variable amounts. This is an example of an assay procedure that should not be *too* specific. The question now remains: Should the metabolites be co-assayed or not? Unfortunately this question cannot be answered decisively, since there are no data available about the activity of the metabolites in man. However, these metabolites are usually present in serum of patients treated with QD. In fig. 5 the results of a method giving only the sum of unchanged QD and DHQD (Armand and Badinand 1972) are plotted against the results of a procedure (Osinga and de Wolff 1976) with which all cinchona alkaloids, that is QD, DHQD and their metabolites, are determined in serum. There is a good correlation between the two methods, which means that in patients there is a fixed ratio between unchanged drugs and metabolites. Approximately fifty percent of the total consists of the more polar metabolites. Thus we see that there is a good correlation between the representatives of both types of assays. We feel

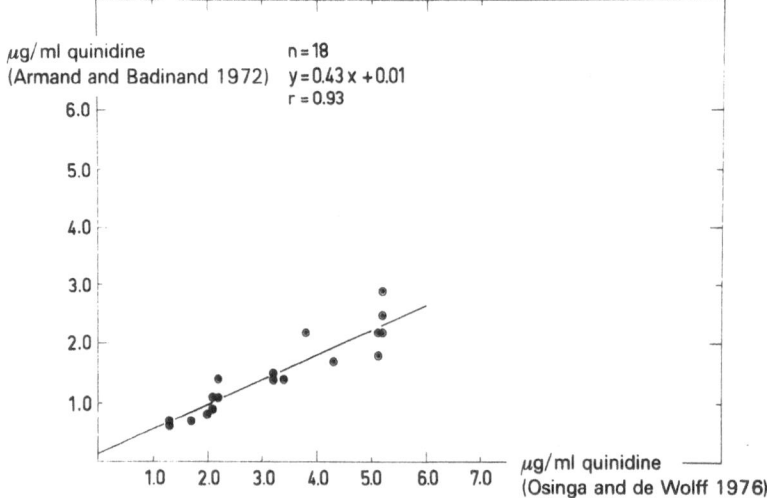

Figure 5. Relationship between the methods of Armand and Badinand (1972) and Osinga and de Wolff (1976) for the determination of quinidine. The former gives only quinidine and dihydro-quinidine; the latter in addition includes the (Active or non-active?) metabolites.

that, in general, it does not make much difference which is chosen. However, for each of these groups of methods a different therapeutic range should be given. For the methods giving QD plus DHQD (Type B) a range of 2–5 mg/l is acceptable, and for methods (Type A) giving the total amount of cinchona alkaloids, thus the metabolites included, a range of 3–8 mg/l suffices. Type C methods should not be used as the contribution of DHQD to the antiarrhythmic effect is neglected. Once again, since no extensive clinical studies on establishing the therapeutic range have been described, the ranges given here must be considered as tentative (table 2).

In the case of patients with impaired hepatic or renal function, the Type A method should not be used alone, since in hepatic disease the relative amount of the metabolites may be decreased, and in patients with renal failure the metabolites may accumulate (Kessler et al. 1974). Therefore the use of both methods will give information about the individual drug metabolism of the patient. When more is known about the relationship between serum levels and clinical effect, and about the activity of the metabolites, a definite choice of "what" and "how what" should be assayed can be made. I assume that this will be a chromatographic procedure giving the concentrations of QD, DHQD and metabolites separately.

PROTEIN BINDING

In patients with renal disease there is another complicating factor. Normally, QD is 70–80 percent bound to plasma proteins. The so-called free or un-bound fraction of 25 percent is generally considered to be the pharmaco-logically active part of the drug. In some patients with impaired renal function, the protein-bound fraction decreases, and as a result the active, non-bound fraction increases (Pérez-Mateo and Erill 1977). Since it is usually the total amount of bound plus unbound drug that is determined, in renal patients symptoms of toxicity may occur at apparently safe serum levels. In the future in such cases the separate determination of bound and unbound fraction may be helpful. For PA, no significant effect of uraemia

Table 2. Tentative therapeutic ranges for quinidine

Method type[a]	Serum concentration (mg/l)
A	3–8
B	2–5
C[b]	–

a. See note at table 1.
b. This method type should not be used since it does not include the active contaminant dihydroquinidine.

on the free fraction is expected, since this drug is only 15 percent bound to plasma proteins.

SAMPLING: WHAT AND WHEN

The problem of protein binding leads us to the question what kind of sample should be taken for drug analysis. The concentration of some drugs in saliva reflects the unbound fraction in plasma, and assays in saliva have been suggested as a tool in clinical practice (Danhof and Breimer 1978). For QD, a correlation between saliva concentrations and total plasma levels could be demonstrated in three subjects (Jaffe et al. 1975). For PA, a little more is known. The secretion of PA into saliva appears to be dependent of saliva pH and it was therefore concluded that measurement of PA concentrations in saliva is not a useful method for monitoring the plasma concentration of PA in patients (Koup et al. 1975). Contradictory to this are the findings of Galeazzi, Benet et al. (1976), who found that saliva concentrations more precisely mirror the therapeutic effect than do plasma levels. These data on the value of saliva concentrations for QD or PA therapy are still scanty and contradictory, and therefore, serum or plasma is, for the time being, the material of choice for the assays of these drugs.

The time for taking blood samples is critical, because these drugs have a relatively short half-life. Since it takes approximately four half-lives to reach a steady-state serum concentration, blood samples for QD or PA assay should be taken one day after the commencement of the therapy. Two samples should then be taken: one just before the first morning dose, and one two hours thereafter. The two values thus found indicate the lower and upper limit of the concentration range of the patient. If the peak level is too high and the lower is in the therapeutic range, then smaller doses should be given more frequently. When both concentrations are too low or too high, the dose should be adjusted before the frequency is changed. Thanks to the development of sustained release preparations, serum concentrations of patients taking QD or PA can be kept in the therapeutic range quite easily. The therapeutically equivalent Kiditard ® and Quinidine Durettes ® can be prescribed twice daily (Soeterboek and van Thiel 1976), and Procainamide Durettes ® three times daily. This is an important improvement as compared to the four-to-six-times-daily prescriptions with the classical formulations.

Once the dose is optimally fixed, it is not necessary to repeat the assay more often than once in two or three months. In this situation, it is usually sufficient to measure the serum concentration just before the first morning dose. In the case of inadequate effect or suspected intoxication, or in the case of a change in the condition of the patient, the determination should be performed more frequently.

CONCLUSIONS

The determination of procainamide (PA) and quinidine (QD) concentrations is a useful tool for antiarrhythmic therapy. Serum is the material of choice for these assays. For PA, a colourimetric method giving only PA concentrations is usually sufficient. In some instances, e.g. in renal impairment, the additional assay of the active metabolite, NAPA, may give relevant information. The generally accepted therapeutic range for PA is 4–8 mg/l. Determination of the acetylator status of the patient may be of prognostic value for the dosage schedule and the occurrence of side effects.

For the monitoring of QD therapy, a fluorometric assay with which all cinchona alkaloids are determined usually suffices. The therapeutic range is then 3–8 mg/l. In patients with impairment of hepatic or renal function, an additional assay of QD plus dihydroquinidine (DHQD) should be performed. For this procedure a therapeutic range of 2–5 mg/l is estimated.

REFERENCES

Ambler, P.K. and Masarei, J.R.L., A new fluorimetric method for procainamide. *Clin Chim. Acta* 70, 379–383 (1976).

Armand, J. and Badinand, A., Dosage de la quinidine (ou de la quinine) dans les milieux biologiques. *Ann. Biol. Clin.* 30, 599–604 (1972).

Atkinson, A.J., Parker, M. and Strong, J. Rapid gas chromatographic measurement of plasma procainamide concentration. *Clin. Chem.* 18, 643–646 (1972).

Bratton, A.C. and Marshall, E.K., A new coupling component for sulfanilamide determination. *J. Biol. Chem.* 128, 537–550 (1939).

Brodie, B.B. and Udenfriend, S., The estimation of quinine in human plasma with a note on the estimation of quinidine. *J. Pharmacol. Exptl. Therap.* 78, 154–158 (1943).

Carr, K., Woosley, R.L. and Oates, J.A., Simultaneous quantification of procainamide and N-acetylprocainamide with high-performance liquid chromatography. *J. Chromatog.* 129, 363–368 (1976).

Christiansen, J., Quantitative *in situ* thin-layer chromatography of quinidine and salicylic acid in capillary blood. *J. Chromatog.* 123, 57–63 (1976).

Conn, H.L. and Luchi, R.J., Some cellular and metabolic considerations relating to the action of quinidine as a prototype antiarrhythmic agent. *Am. J. Med.* 37, 685–699 (1964).

Cramér, G. and Isaksson, B., Quantitative determination of quinidine in plasma. *Scandinav. J. Clin. Lab. Investigation* 15, 553–556 (1963).

Crouthamel, W.G., Kowarski, B. and Narang, P.K., Specific serum quinidine assay by high-performance liquid chromatography. *Clin. Chem.* 23, 2030–2033 (1977).

Danhof, M. and Breimer, D.D., Therapeutic drug monitoring in saliva. *Clin. Pharmacokin.* 3, 39–57 (1978).

Drayer, D.E., Lowenthal, D.T., Woosley, R.L., Nies, A.S., Schwartz, A. and Reidenberg,

M.M., Cumulation of N-acetylprocainamide, an active metabolite of procainamide, in patients with impaired renal function. *Clin. Pharmacol. Therap.* 22, 63–69 (1977).

Drayer, D.E., Reidenberg, M.M. and Sevy, R.W., N-acetylprocainamide: an active metabolite of procainamide. *Proc. Soc. Exptl. Biol. Med.* 146, 358–363 (1974).

Dutcher, J.S. and Strong, J.M., Determination of plasma procainamide and N-acetylprocainamide concentration by high-pressure liquid chromatography. *Clin. Chem.* 23, 1318–1320 (1977).

Elevitch, F.R., *Fluorometric Techniques in Clinical Chemistry*, Boston, 1973, pp. 154–159.

Evans, D.A.P., An improved and simplified method of detecting the acetylator phenotype. *J. Med. Genet.* 6, 405–407 (1969).

Frey, W., Über Vorhofflimmern beim Menschen und seine Beseitigung durch Chinidin. *Berl. Klin. Wschr.* 55, 450–452 (1918A).

Frey, W., Weitere Erfahrungen mit Chinidin bei absoluter Herzunregelmässigkeit. *Berl. Klin. Wschr.* 55, 849–853 (1918B).

Frislid, K., Berg, M., Hansteen, V. and Lunde, P.K.M., Comparison of the acetylation of procainamide and sulfadimidine in man. *Europ. J. Clin. Pharmacol.* 9, 433–438 (1976).

Frislid, K., Bredesen, J.E. and Lunde, P.K.M., Fluorometric or gas-liquid chromatographic determination of procainamide? *Clin. Chem.* 21, 1180–1182 (1975).

Galeazzi, R.L., Benet, L.Z. and Sheiner, L.B., Relationship between the pharmacokinetics and pharmacodynamics of procainamide. *Clin. Pharmacol. Ther.* 20, 278–289 (1976).

Galeazzi, R.L., Sheiner, L.B., Lockwood, T. and Benet, L.Z., The renal elimination of procainamide. *Clin. Pharmacol. Therap.* 19, 55–62 (1976).

Gey, G.O., Levy, R.H., Pettet, G. and Fisher, L., Quinidine plasma concentration and exertional arrhythmia. *Am. Heart J.* 90, 19–24 (1975).

Gibson, T.P., Lowenthal, D.T., Nelson, H.A. and Briggs, W.A., Elimination of procainamide in end stage renal failure. *Clin. Pharmacol. Therap.* 17, 321–329 (1975).

Gibson, T.P., Matusik, J., Matusik, E., Nelson, H.A., Wilkinson, J. and Briggs, W.A., Acetylation of procainamide in man and its relationship to isonicotinic acid hydrazide. acetylation phenotype. *Clin. Pharmacol. Therap.* 17, 395–399 (1975).

Härtel, G. and Harjanne, A., Comparison of two methods for quinidine determination and chromatographic analysis of the difference. *Clin. Chim. Acta* 23, 289–294 (1969).

Hamfelt, A. and Malers, E., Determination of quinidine concentration in serum in the control of quinidine therapy. *Acta. Soc. Med. Uppsal.* 68, 181–191 (1963).

Huffman, D.H. and Hignite, C.E., Serum quinidine concentrations: comparison of fluorescence, gas-chromatographic, and gas-chromatographic/mass-spectrometric methods. *Clin. Chem.* 22, 810–812 (1976).

Jaffe, J.M., Strum, J.D., Martineau, P.C. and Colaizzi, J.L., Relationship between quinidine plasma and saliva levels in humans. *J. Pharm. Sci.* 64, 2028–2029 (1975).

Karlsson, E., Clinical pharmacokinetics of procainamide. *Clin. Pharmacokin.* 3, 97–107 (1978).

Kessler, K.M., Lowenthal, D.T., Warner, H., Gibson, T., Briggs, W. and Reidenberg, M.M., Quinidine elimination in patients with congestive heart failure or poor renal function. *New Engl. J. Med.* 290, 706–709 (1974).

Koch-Weser, J., Serum procainamide levels as therapeutic guides. *Clin. Pharmacokin.* 2, 389–403 (1977).

Koch-Weser, J. and Klein, S.W., Procainamide dosage schedules, plasma concentrations, and clinical effects. *J. Am. Med. Ass.* 215, 1454–1460 (1971).

Koup, J.R., Jusko, W.J., and Goldfarb, A.L., pH-Dependent secretion of procainamide into saliva. *J. Pharm. Sci.* 64, 2008–2010 (1975).

Kutsch Lojenga, J.C., Kinidine-bepaling in serum/plasma. *Mededelingen Groep van Ziekenhuisapothekers* 28, 21–23 (1972).

Lima, J.J. and Jusko, W.J., Determination of procainamide acetylator status. *Clin. Pharmacol. Ther.* 23, 25–29 (1978).

Lunde, P.K.M., Frislid, K. and Hansteen, V., Disease and acetylation polymorphism. *Clin. Pharmacokin.* 2, 182–197 (1977).

Midha, K.K. and Charette, C., GLC determination of quinidine from plasma and whole blood. *J. Pharm. Sci.* 63, 1244–1247 (1974).

Moulin, M.A. and Kinsun, H., A gas-liquid chromatographic method for quantitative determination of quinidine in blood. *Clin. Chim. Acta* 75, 491–495 (1977).

Mulder, C. and Faber, D.B., Een bepalingsmethode voor kinidine en hydrokinidine in plasma. *Pharm. Weekbl.* 108, 289–293 (1973).

Osinga, A. and de Wolff, F.A., Determination of quindine in human serum in the presence of diuretics. *Clin. Chim. Acta* 73, 505–512 (1976).

Pérez-Mateo, M. and Erill, S., Protein binding of salicylate and quinidine in plasma from patients with renal failure, chronic liver disease and chronic respiratory insufficiency. *Europ. J. Clin. Pharmacol.* 11, 225–231 (1977).

Powers, J.L. and Sadee, W., Determination of quinidine by high-performance liquid chromatography. *Clin. Chem.* 24, 299–302 (1978).

Refsum, H., Frislid, K., Lunde, P.K.M. and Landmark, K.H., Effects of N-acetylprocainamide as compared with procainamide in isolated rat atria. *Eur. J. Pharmacol.* 33, 47–52 (1975).

Rocco, R.M., Abbott, D.C., Giese, R.W., and Karger, B.L., Analysis for procainamide and N-acetylprocainamide in plasma or serum by high-performance liquid chromatography. *Clin. Chem.* 23, 705–708 (1977).

Scott, C.G., Anderson, R.C. and Chen, K.K., Comparison of the pharmacologic action of quinidine and dihydroquinidine. *J. Pharmacol. Exptl. Therap.* 84, 184–188 (1945).

Shukur, L.R., Powers, J.L., Marques, R.A., Winter, M.E., and Sadee, W., Measurement of procainamide and N-acetylprocainamide in serum by high-performance liquid chromatography. *Clin. Chem.* 23, 636–638 (1977).

Sitar, D. S., Graham, D.N., Rangno, R.E., Dusfresne, L.R., and Ogilvie, R.I., Modified colorimetric method for procainamide in plasma. *Clin. Chem.* 22, 379–380 (1976).

Sjöqvist, F., Borgå, O. and Orme, M.L'E. Fundamentals of Clinical Pharmacology. In: *Drug Treatment*. Ed., Avery, G.S., Sydney 1976 p. 32.

Sloman, J.G., Cardiovascular Diseases. In: *Drug Treatment*. Ed., Avery, G.S., Sydney, 1976, p. 450ff.

Soeterboek, A.M. and van Thiel, M., Serum quinidine levels after chronic administration of four different quinidine formulations. *J. Int. Med. Res.* 4, 393–401 (1976).

Sterling, J., Cox, S. and Haney, W.G., Comparison of procainamide analyses in plasma by spectrophotofluorometry, colorimetry and GLC. *J. Pharm. Sci.* 63, 1744–1747 (1974).

Steyn, J.M. and Hundt, H.K.L., A thin-layer chromatographic method for the quantitative determination of quinidine in human serum. *J. Chromatog.* 111, 463–465 (1975).

Valentine, J.L., Driscoll, P., Hamburg, E.L., and Thompson, E.D., GLC Determination of quinidines in human plasma. *J. Pharm. Sci.* 65, 96–98 (1976).

Weddle, O.H. and Mason W.D., Rapid determination of procainamide and its N-acetyl derivative in human plasma by high-pressure liquid chromatography. *J. Pharm. Sci.* 66, 874–875 (1977).

Wesley-Hadzija, B. and Mattocks, A.M., Quantitative thin-layer chromatographic method for the determination of procainamide and its major metabolite in plasma. *J. Chromatog.* 143, 307–313 (1977).

14. LIDOCAINE

H. WESSELING

Over the last twenty years, lidocaine has become increasingly popular as a first-line drug for the treatment of cardiac arrhythmias of ventricular origin. In particular rhythm disturbances due to acute myocardial infarction form the main indications for the use of this drug, either alone – ventricular ectopic beats, VEBs – or following direct current cardio-version – ventricular tachycardia, ventricular fibrillation (Gianelly et al. 1967; Harrison and Alderman 1970; Lown, 1966; Pitt et al. 1971; Southworth et al. 1950; Wyman 1974) – see table 1.

Plasma levels of the drug that are considered to prevent or effectively suppress VEBs lie between 1.2 and 6.0 μg/ml. This range was originally determined by administering lidocaine in varying doses by intravenous injection to patients with VEBs (Gianelly et al. 1967). The range between plasma concentrations that do not suppress VEBs and concentrations that exert toxic effects on the central nervous system was defined as the range of effective concentrations. There is not much wrong with this method, except that it does not always seem to work. Unwanted symptoms may occur even at lower plasma levels (table 2), whereas on the other hand plasma levels that are considered to be effective do not always prevent or suppress VEBs. This will be discussed later.

Nevertheless, various techniques of administration have been developed with the aim of rapid achievement and long-lasting maintenance of these so-called effective plasma levels (table 3).

Intravenous constant infusion at a rate of 1.5–3.5 mg/min or 20–50 μg/kg of body weight per minute will produce plasma levels between 1.5 and 5 μg/ml (Boyes 1971). For each drug that is given by i.v. infusion it will take about three half-lives before approximately ninety percent of the steady-

Table 1. Emergency treatment of ventricular arrhythmias.

VEBs	1	2	3
VEBs	lidocaine	disopyramide procainamide	DPH
tachycardia	cardio-version	lidocaine	procainamide
fibrillation	cardio-version	external massage	cardio-version and lidocaine or β-blockers

Table 2. Unwanted lidocaine effects with increasing blood levels.

μg/ml $\longrightarrow$	3	5	7	9	11 and >
CNS	dizziness drowsiness euphoria paresthesias	confusion excitement speech disturbed muscle fasciculations nausea, vomiting	seizures	coma	
TC, TR	↑ pulse rate (slight) B.P		hypotension bradycardia	respiratory arrest	

Table 3. Various possible lidocaine dose regimens.

Route	Dose regimen	Advantages and disadvantages
Intravenous	Continuous infusion, 2–3 mg/min	Takes hours before steady state is reached
	One or more boluses, followed by continuous infusion	
	Loading infusion (continuous infusion with decreasing concentration)	No "dip" after bolus
Intramuscular	200–300 mg	Early prevention
	200–300 mg., followed by continuous infusion	give in deltoid muscle, beware bradycardia
Orally	250–500 mg	Not effective More toxicity (??)

state concentration is obtained. Since lidocaine has a half-life (β-phase) in man of roughly two hours, one may expect that only after about six hours will this 90-percent level be obtained. In modern practice therefore, lidocaine therapy is started with a bolus injection of 75–100 mg (Rydén et al. 1973), two small boluses within 10 minutes, or a loading infusion (Greenblatt et al. 1976), both followed by continuous i.v. infusion at a rate of 2–3 mg/kg for 24 hours or more. Some clinicians diminish the infusion rate gradually over several hours (Aps et al. 1976).

It is well documented that most people who die from ventricular fibrillation due to acute myocardial infarction, do so in the very first hours after the beginning of the symptoms of infarction (Lie et al. 1976; Partridge and Geddes 1970 Vonk 1971). The intramuscular injection of lidocaine in doses between 200–400 mg, either by the family doctor, ambulance personnel, or even the patient himself (if a high-risk individual) has been strongly advocated (Dunning et al. 1973; Fehmers and Dunning 1972; Martin 1970; Rydén et al. 1973, 1975; Shen and Kocot 1976; Sheridan et al. 1977; Valentine et al. 1974); this can be followed by continuous i.v. infusion (Shen and Gibaldi 1974). The injections should be given into the deltoid muscle (Cohen et al. 1970; Meyer and Zelechowski 1970; Schwartz et al. 1974; Zener et al. 1973); most authors claim that this will cause peak plasma levels within fifteen minutes, that, again, fall in the effective concentration range.

Oral administration of lidocaine should be very attractive, due to its ease and to its preventive potential. Since the liver extracts approximately seventy percent of the lidocaine from the portal circulation during the first passage (Stenson et al. 1971), the amount of unchanged drug that reaches the general circulation after oral administration is very small (Boyes 1971; Keenaghan and Boyes 1972; Scott et al 1970). No effect on VEBs after oral administration of 250–500 mg was observed (Fehners and Durring 1972); whether the accumulation of metabolites results in ineffectiveness or toxicity remains to be seen: this will be discussed later.

Since the development of reliable and sensitive gas chromatographic methods (Keenaghan, 1968), plasma levels of lidocaine can easily be followed and computer techniques that predict steady-state plasma levels based on body-weight and cardiac output data may provide the cardiologist with perfect guidelines for his dosage regime (Greenblatt et al. 1976: Jeliffe et al. 1975).

The main problems that seem to threaten the therapist are variations in the patient's condition that may influence the plasma levels, i.e. "effective concentrations" (table 4).

Table 4. Factors that may influence the effects of lidocaine.

Complication	Lidocaine	Effect	Comments
Heart failure	↑	↑ or =	Vd ↓, bad perfusion
Liver blood flow decreased	↑	↑	Decreased metabolism
Renal failure	=	=	Toxic metabs ↑ (?)
K^+ ↓	=	↓	Membrane susceptibility ↑
Digitalis			Ibid.
Acidosis	↑	↑	Vd ↓, ionization ↑
Higher concentration	free ↑	↑	Protein binding ↓

Of course the infarction may seriously affect cardiac output and thus the blood flow to various organs. This may in general lead to a smaller volume of distribution, i.e. higher blood levels, whereas impairment of liver blood flow will cause a decrease in metabolic clearance (Stenson et al. 1971; Thomson et al. 1973). In these cases dosage should be appropriately adapted, and sometimes halved.

Changes in glomerular filtration rate do not affect the elimination of lidocaine to a great extent, since renal excretion does not contribute more than approximately ten percent to total clearance (Eriksson et al. 1966). The removal of more polar metabolites, however, may be impaired.

Other changes in the patients internal milieu may influence either lidocaine kinetics or dynamics to some degree, though the relevance of this influence is not always clear. Potassium depletion will render the myocardial cell membrane more sensitive, i.e. arrhythmias may arise more frequently; the same is true for digitalized patients and in both cases lidocaine may be less effective (Bigger and Giardina 1974; Thomson 1974). Acidosis may lead to a higher proportion of ionized lidocaine (pKa = 7.85) and thus to a smaller volume of distribution and to higher plasma levels (Hayes 1970). High plasma concentrations of lidocaine are relatively less protein-bound and therefore their activity may be slightly underestimated (Tucker et al. 1970).

Interactions with other drugs may play a role (table 5): enzyme inducers (barbiturates) are known to shorten lidocaine half-life (Heinonen et al. 1970); propranolol may reduce, by its cardiodepressive effect, the volume of distribution, and in a pharmacodynamic sense, it may also add to the anti-arrhythmic effect of lidocaine; (Branch et al. 1973) β-adrenergic stimulants like isoproterenol will have the reverse effect (Benowitz et al. 1974). Morphine is said to increase cerebral blood flow and thus to augment central nervous toxicity (Miller et al. 1972); on the other hand, as we could demonstrate in mice, opioid drugs suppress lidocaine-induced convulsions very effectively, though they do not reduce mortality (Wesseling 1972).

With regard to the various influences mentioned above and by adjusting, if necessary, the dose accordingly, it must theoretically be possible to

Table 5. Interactions of lidocaine with other drugs.

Drug	Lidocaine	Effect	Comment
Barbiturates	↓	↓	Increased metabolism
Propranolol		↑	Vd↓, additive pharmacodynamic effect
Catecnolamines	depends	depends	Vd↓ or ↑ membrane susceptibility
Opiates	CNS ↑	?	central blood flow ↑
	Heart ↑		toxicity ↓ (?)

obtain any desired plasma level of lidocaine in an individual patient. However, the crucial question is: *are we sure that the desired blood level is the (most) effective blood level* (Halkin 1974)? Most workers, though not all (Bleifeld et al. 1973; Darby et al. 1972; Gamble and Cohn 1972), find that lidocaine in the recommended concentrations will depress VEBs. But some of them found that the rate of ventricular fibrillation (Chopra et al. 1971; Darby et al. 1972; Lie et al. 1973) or death-rate in general (Lie et al. 1974; Pitt et al. 1971) did not differ between lidocaine-treated and placebo-treated groups of patients.

It may be possible that arrhythmias that are really dangerous are not, or not sufficiently, suppressed in some patients. This may especially be true for arrhythmias that arise immediately at the onset of the infarction and that are responsible for the majority of fatal issues (Pantridge 1970). If that is so, one may doubt whether repeated intravenous injections of 100 mg lidocaine combined with 200–300 mg intramuscularly as a first-aid measure, as is recommended in the Netherlands (Vonk 1971) does decrease death rate due to ventricular fibrillation. It seems to me a wise policy to give this therapy the benefit of the doubt and to wait for further results of prospective studies concerned with this problem.

Another major complication is that it is still uncertain how far a "dangerous" (or "warning") arrhythmia really is predictive of the onset of ventricular fibrillation (Lie et al. 1973). It may be that bursts of ventricular tachycardial attacks are the best indication (Loefmark and Orinius 1977), or, in chronic situations, the occurrence of ectopics with short RR' intervals (Ruberman et al. 1977).

In studies that might throw more light on this problem a careful analysis of those irregularities that precede a fibrillatory attack *combined* with plasma level measurements in that individual is required as soon as possible. They may perhaps lead to the prevention of elaborate infusion systems that give splendid but useless plasma levels against innocent VEBs.

Related to the problem of which abnormal ventricular beats we should treat are the questions whether too low blood levels may be harmful and whether steady state is really the most desirable condition. There is evidence that lidocaine in low concentrations may promote re-entry phenomena and thus cause rhythm disturbances (Gamble and Cohn 1972; Geddes et al. 1972; Sasyniuk and Ogilvie 1975). In this light one may ask whether the low levels found after subcutaneous local anaesthesia, used for catheterization, (Schwartz 1974), are really "ineffective".

Alderman et al. (1974) found that in the presence of "effective" plasma levels small boluses could effectively suppress hitherto resistant VEBs, suggesting that Δ-concentration does the job, as it were by a sort of pharmacological defibrillation.

In this respect it is noteworthy that in laboratory animals the ratio myocardial-plasma concentration of lidocaine under steady-state conditions was found to be practically unity. After five to fifteen minutes following a bolus injection, however, this ratio is in rats much greater than unity (fig. 1). In the light of these considerations we initiated, in cooperation with the cardiology department of the St. Anthonius Hospital and the Medical Physical Institute (MFI) in Utrecht a clinical study in which i.v. and bolus injections will be compared in their effect on various types of VEBs, with special attention to changes in RR'-intervals and concomitant plasma levels.

Finally, the possible role of metabolites should be elucidated in more detail. Two dealkylated metabolites, mono-ethyl-glycine-xylidide (MEGX) and glycine-xylidide (GX) are known to occur in man (Halkin et al. 1975), and perhaps a ring-hydroxylated product, metahydroxylidocaine (MHL), apart from glucuronated derivatives. Since both MEGX and GX are weaker convulsants and antiarrhythmics than the parent drug in animal models (Blumer et al. 1973; Smith and Duce 1971), it is doubtful whether they contribute to the wanted and unwanted activities of lidocaine to any great extent, especially after the single doses used in oral studies. After long-term infusions however, they may accumulate due to their rather long half-lives, especially GX (Halkin et al. 1975; Strong et al. 1975), and estimation of their plasma levels is then desirable. We found gas chromatographic detection of lidocaine, MEGX, GX and MHL in one sample difficult, even after derivatization, because of the poor recovery of the polar metabolites (Tan, i.p.).

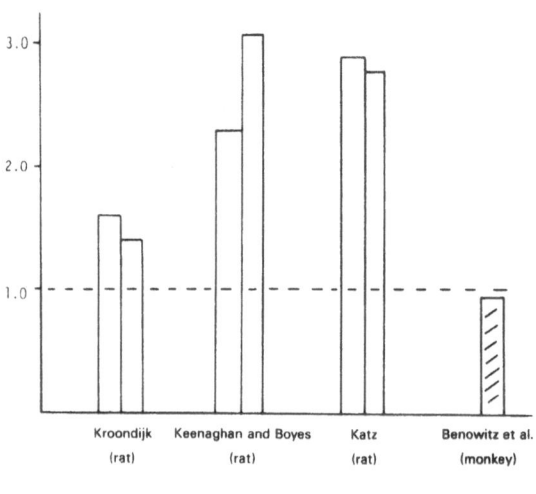

left column: after 5'
right column: after 15'
hatched column: steady state

Figure 1. Myocardial plasma concentration coefficients of lidocaine after bolus injections and under steady-state conditions for laboratory animals (Kroondijk 1977; Keenaghar and Boyes 1972; Katz 1968; Berowitz et al. 1974).

High-pressure liquid chromatography techniques will be required for a reliable determination of all metabolites in one sample, so that a "weighed" activity can be estimated.

As was shown in table 2, minor symptoms of CNS toxicity are frequently seen and occasionally major events (convulsions) may occur (Pfeifer et al. 1976). In the majority of cases, discontinuing the infusion will be sufficient to abolish these symptoms; if anticonvulsant therapy is needed we would, based on animal studies, recommend diazepam rather than a barbiturate (Wesseling 1972).

Quaternary lidocaine derivatives recently developed (Kniffer et al. 1974) do not seem to be of great advantage to us, since signs of CNS toxicity will be obscured and circulatory disturbances may suddenly appear.

In conclusion we may say that lidocaine does suppress VEBs after myocardial infarction in the majority of cases, though it is not clear whether it suppresses all, and especially "dangerous", arrhythmias.

Runs of VEBs, multifocal beats, bigeminal rhythm, and the occurrence of three to five and more VEBs per minute are indications for giving lidocaine: at home 1.5 mg/kg i.v., repeated once or twice after ten minutes if necessary, and/or 3–4 mg/kg into the deltoid muscle. In the coronary case unit two bolus injections of 1 mg/kg given over a one-minute period, separated by a ten minute interval and followed by a constant infusion of 2–3 mg/min for 24–36 hours are recommended.

Further studies on the nature and treatment of dangerous arrhythmias, on bolus kinetics and dynamics and on the role of metabolites may close still-existing gaps in our knowledge about this important drug.

REFERENCES

Alderman, E.L., Kerber, R.E. and Harrison, D.C. *Am. J. Cardiol.* 34, 342–349 (1974).
Aps, C., Bell, J.A., Jenkins, B.S., et al., *Brit. Med. J.*, Jan. 3, 13–15 (1976).
Benowitz, N., Forsyth, R.P., Melmon, K.L., et al., *Clin. Pharmacol. Ther.*, 16, 1, 87–109 (1974).
Bigger, J.T., Jr. and Giardina, E.G.V., In: *Cardiovascular Drug Therapy*. Ed. Melmon K., Philadelphia, 1974, p. 104 ff.
Bleifeld, W., Merx, W., Heinrich, K.W., et al., *Eur. J. Clin. Pharmacol.* 6, 119–126 (1973).
Blumer, J., Strong, J.M. and Atkinson, A.J., *J. Pharmacol. Expt Ther.* 186, 31–36 (1973).
Boyes, R.N., *J. Clin. Pharmacol. Ther.* 12, 1, 105–117 (1971).
Branch, R.A., Shand, D.G., Wilkinson G., et al., *J. Pharmacol. Expt. Ther.* 184, 515–519 (1973).
Chopra, M.P., Thadani, V., Portal, R.W., et al., *Br. Med. J.* 3, 668 (1971).
Cohen, L.S., Atkins, J.M., Matthew, O.A., et al., *Circulation* 41–42, Suppl. 3, 537 (1970).
Darby, S., Bennett, M.A., Cruickshank, J.C., et al., *Lancet*, April, 817–819 (1972).
Dunning, A.J., Roos, J.C. and Fehmers, M.C.O., *Neth. J. Med.* 16, 178–188 (1973).
Eriksson, E., Granberg, P.O. and Ortengren, B., *Acta Chir. Scand.* 358, 55–69 (1966).
Fehmers, M.C.O. and Dunning, A.J., *Am. J. Cardiol.* 29, 514 (1972).
Fehmers, M.C.O., van Daatselaar, J.J. and Dunning, A.J., *N.T.v. Gen.* 116, 29, 1214–1220 (1972).
Gamble, O.W. and Cohn, K., *Circulation*, 46, 498–506 (1972).
Geddes, J.S., Webb., S.W. and Pantridge, J.F., *Brit. Heart J.* 34, 964 (1972).

Gianelly, R., von der Groeben, J.O., Spivack, A.P. and Harrison, D.C., *N. Eng. J. Med.* 277, 1215 (1967).

Greenblatt, J., et al., *J.A.M.A.* 236, 3, 273–277 (1976).

Halkin, H., In: *Cardiovascular Drug Therapy.* Ed., Melmon, K., Philadelphia, 1974, p. 120 ff.

Halkin, H., Meffin, P., Melmon, K.L. and Rowland, M., *Clin. Pharmacol. Ther.* 17, 6, 669–676 (1975).

Harrison, D.C. and Alderman, E.L., In: *Lidocaine in the Treatment of Ventricular Arrhythmias.* Ed., Scott, D.B. and Julian, D.G., Edinburgh, 1970, pp. 178–188.

Hayes, A.H., In: *Lidocaine in the Treatment of Ventricular Arrhythmias.* Ed., Scott, D.B. and Julian, D.G., Edinburgh, 1970, pp. 189–199.

Heinonen, J., Takki, S. and Jarho, L., *Acta Anaesth. Scand.* 14, 89–95 (1970).

Jeliffe, R., Guicoechea, F., Tuey, D., et al., *Clin. Res.* 13, 125A (1975).

Katz, J., *Anesthesiology* 253 (1968).

Keenaghan, J.B., *Anesthesiology* 29, 110–112 (1968).

Keenaghan, J.B. and Boyes, R.N., *J. Pharmacol. Exp. Ther.* 180, 454–463 (1972).

Kniffen, F.J., Lomas, T.E., Nobel-Allen, N.L., et al., *Circulation* 49, 264–271 (1974).

Kroondijk, T., "Relationship lidocaine kinetics and effect." Unpublished results, 1977.

Lie, K.I., Wellens, H.J., van Capelle, F.J., et al., *N. Eng. J. Med.* 291, 1329–1326 (1974).

Lie, K.L., Wellens, H.J.J., Downar, E., et al., *Circulation* 54, 845 (1976).

Lie, K.I., Wellens, H.J. and Durrer, D., *Eur. J. Cardiol.* 1, 379–389 (1973).

Loefmark, R. and Orinius, E., *Acta Med. Scand.* 201, 89–91 (1977).

Lown, B., In: *The Current Status of Intensive Coronary Care.* Philadelphia, 1966, pp. 42–45.

Martin, R.O., *Brit. Med. J.* 2, 513 (1970).

Meyer, M.B. and Zelechowski, K., In: *Lidocaine in the Treatment of Ventricular Arrhythmias.* Ed., Scott, D.B. and Julian, D.G., Edinburgh, 1970; pp. 161–166.

Miller, R.L., Forsyth., R.P. and Melmon, K.L., *Pharmacology* 7, 138 (1972).

Pantridge, J.F., In: *Lidocaine in the Treatment of Ventricular Arrhythmias.* Ed., Scott, D.B. and Julian D.G., Edinburgh, 1970.

Pantridge, J.F. and Geddes, J.S., *Eur. J. Cardiol.* 1, 335 (1974).

Pfeifer, H.J., et al, *Am. Heart J.*, 92, 2, 168–173 (1976).

Pitt, A., Lipp, H. and Anderson, S.T., *Lancet*, March, 612–616 (1971).

Ruberman, W., Weinblatt, E., Goldberg, J.D., et al., *N. Eng. J. Med.* 14, 750–757 (1977).

Rydén, L., Waldenström, A. and Ehn, L., *Br. Heart J.* 35, 1124–1131 (1973).

Rydén, L., Waldenström, A., Winsnes, Y. et al., *Am. Heart. J.* 89, 4 (1975).

Sasyniuk, B.I. and Ogilvie, R.I., *Ann. Rev. Pharmacol.* 131 (1975).

Schwartz, M.L., *Am. Heart J.* 88, 6, 721–723 (1974).

Schwartz, M.L., Meyer, M.B., Covino, B.G., et al., *J. Clin. Pharmacol.* 77–83 (1974).

Scott, D.B., Jebson, P.J., Godman, M.J. and Julian, D.G., *Lancet*, Jan., 193 (1970).

Shen, D. and Gibaldi, M., *J. Clin. Pharmacol.*, July, 339–349 (1974).

Shen, J.B. and Kocot, S.L., *Am. Heart J.* 91, 4, 430–436 (1976).

Sheridan, D.J., Rawlins, M., Crawford, L., et al., *Lancet*, April 16, 824–825 (1977).

Smith, E.B. and Duce, B.R., *J. Pharmacol. Expt. Ther.* 179, 3, 580–586 (1971).

Southworth, J.L., McKusick, V.A., Pierce, E.C., et al., *J.A.M.A.* 199, 156 (1950).

Stenson, R.E., Constantino, R.T. and Harrison, D.E., *Circulation* 43, 205–211 (1971).

Strong, J.M., Mayfield, D.E., Atkinson, A.J., et al., *Clin. Pharmacol. Ther.* 17 184–194 (1975).

Tan, B.H., "Gas Chromatography of Lidocaine and Metabolites." In press.

Thomson, P.D., In: *Cardiovascular Drug Therapy.* Ed., Melmon K., Philadelphia, 1974, p. 60 ff.

Thomson, P.D., Rowland, M., et al., *Ann. Int. Med.* 78, 499–508 (1973).

Tucker, G.T., Boyes, R.N., Bridenbaugh, P.O., et al., *Anesthesiology* 33, 287 (1970).

Valentine, P.A., Frew, J.L., Mashford, M.L., et al., *N. Eng. J. Med.* 291, 1327–1331 (1974).

Vonk, J.T.C., *Huisarts en Wetenschap.* 14, 4 (1971).

Wesseling, H., University thesis, Groningen, 1972.

Wyman, M.G., *Am. J. Cardiol.* 33, 661–667 (1974).

Zener, J.C., Kerber, R.E.. Spivack, A.P.. et al., *Circulation* 47, 984 (1973).

PART III

TOXICOLOGY

15. EPIDEMIOLOGY OF INTOXICATION WITH DRUGS IN AMSTERDAM

H. TIMMERS

Because there is considerable experience of cases of self-poisoning with medicinal drugs in Amsterdam, I investigated the epidemiology of self-intoxication in this city (Timmers 1975). How grave is this problem? Our study, which can no longer be called recent, focused on patients with self-intoxication admitted to the Department of Internal Medicine of the Queen Wilhelmina Hospital over a period of fifteen years, from 1 January 1959 to 1 January 1974. The question may be raised whether this study in a single hospital can yield results which are representative of the whole city, and particularly if the results give any information on the actual incidence of self-intoxication. There is some reason to believe they indeed do so. The municipal health service, which collects these patients from their homes or elsewhere, until very recently made it a rule to transport them to the Queen Wilhelmina Hospital, first of all because our department has an intensive care unit with facilities for artificial ventilation, and secondly

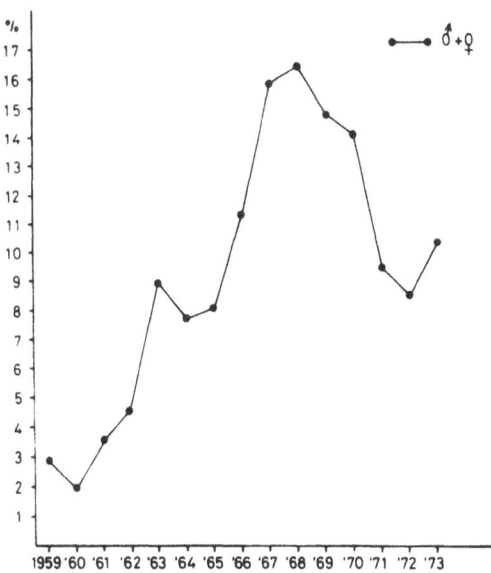

Figure 1. Percentual contribution of admissions for self-intoxication to all admissions to the Department of Internal Medicine of the Queen Wilhelmina Hospital in Amsterdam.

because our hospital has a psychiatric department on its premises, to which
mentally disturbed patients can be transferred if necessary. This policy of the
municipal health service has given us a great deal of work, but on the other
hand it has given us a fairly reliable insight into what happens in Amsterdam
in the field of self-intoxication.

As already mentioned, the study covered a period of fifteen years. The
total number of patients was 1445. Fig. 1 shows that the percentual contribution of self-intoxication to the total number of admissions to the Department of Internal Medicine has markedly increased. In 1959 these cases
accounted for 2.9 percent of all admissions; in 1968 a peak of 16 percent was
reached, which has now dropped to about 10 percent. Smith (1972) reported
a similar figure for the Sheffield area.

Fig. 2 shows the sex distribution, indicating a female predominance in all
years. The same has been observed in foreign series: in Edinburgh (Matthew
and Lawson, 1966); in Sheffield (Smith 1972); and in Brisbane (Baker 1969).
The relative change in admissions for self-intoxication was the same for
both sexes (fig. 3). The mean age of the female patients was higher than that

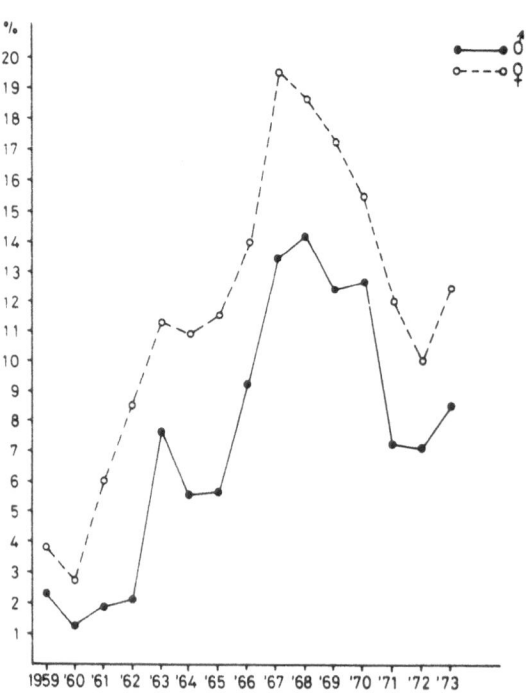

Figure 2. Percentual contributions of admissions of males and females for self-intoxication to all admissions of males and females to the Department of Internal Medicine of the
Queen Wilhelmina Hospital in Amsterdam.

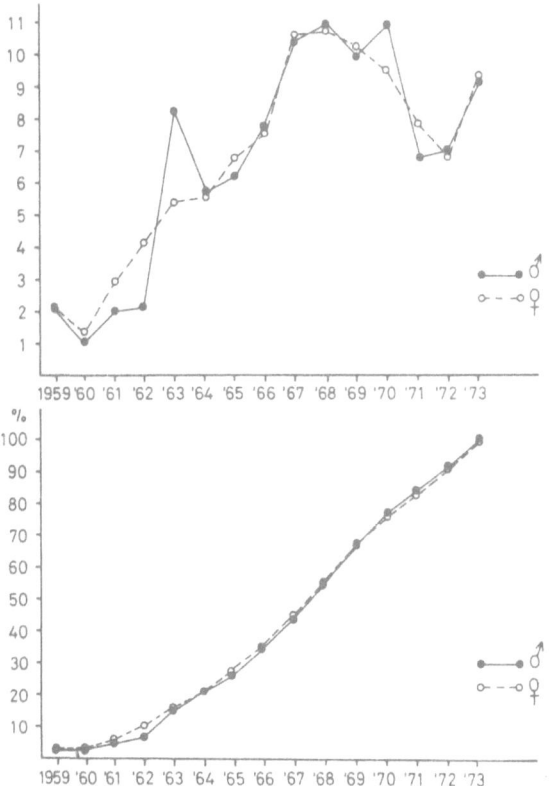

Figure 3. Upper part: percentage per year of male and female patients of the total number of males and females admitted for self-poisoning during the period 1959–1974. Lower part: the same, cumulatively plotted.

of the males, the difference being statistically significant, but in publications from other countries this difference is less marked. The mean age of patients of both sexes decreased during the first years of the study, this being more marked in the males (fig. 4). In the age group under 50 the greatest change occurred in age group 20–30 in the males. This change was less distinct in the females (fig. 5). In both sexes, the decrease in age was virtually the same in the group over 50 (fig. 6). Considering the entire patient population, we find that most patients were in age group 20–30; this again was most conspicuous in the males (fig. 7). It is generally accepted that certain seasons can cause a depression in the human mood. In our series of self-intoxication, however, we found no evidence to this effect (fig. 8). Although the curves suggest peaks and dips, the differences were not statistically significant.

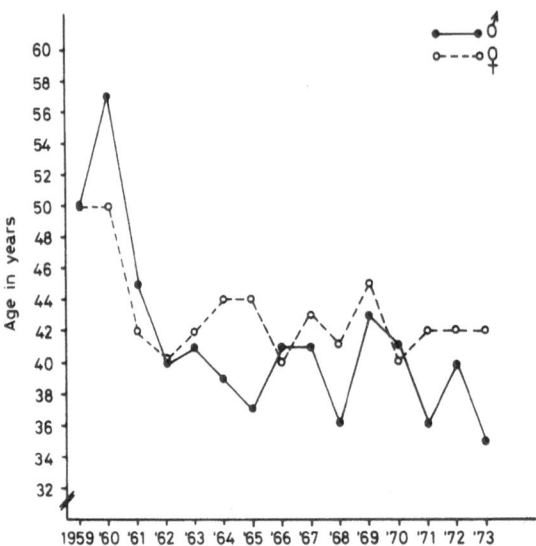

Figure 4. Mean age of male and female self-intoxication patients in each year.

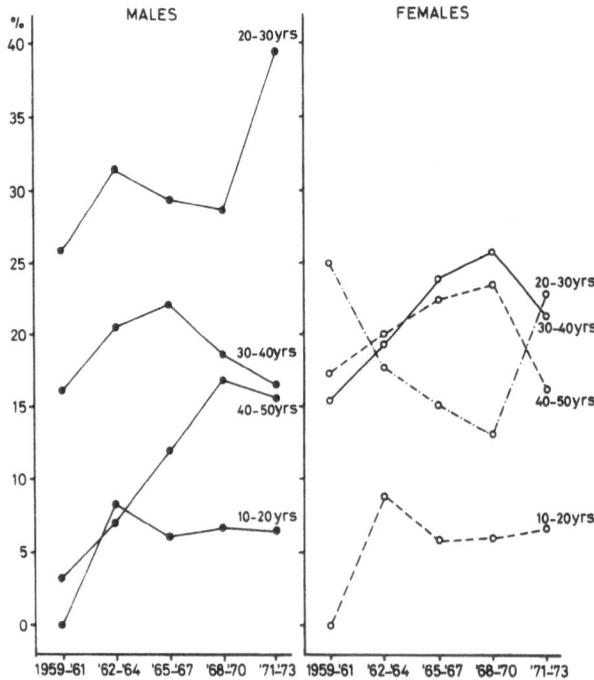

Figure 5. Age-group distribution of self-intoxication admissions (up to 50 years) in three-year periods.

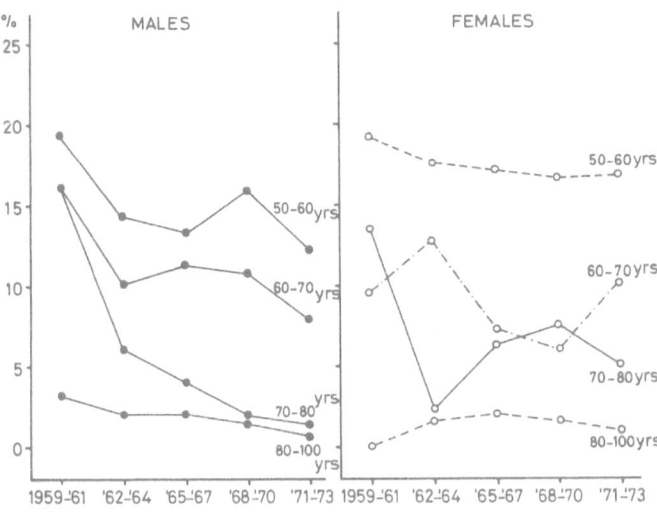

Figure 6. Age-group distribution of self-intoxication admissions (over 50 years) in three-year periods.

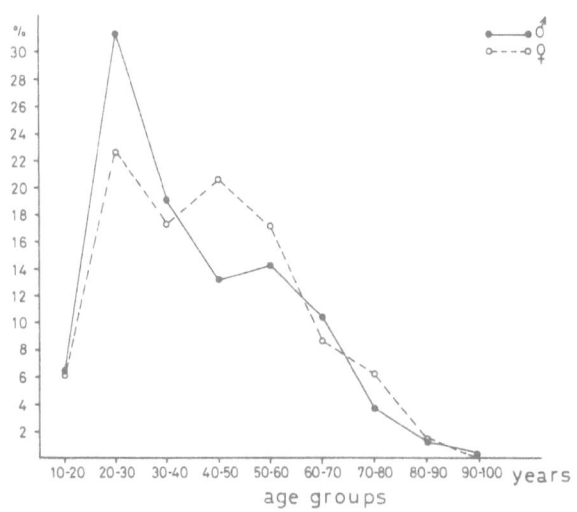

Figure 7. Age-group distribution of self-intoxication admissions throughout the study.

With regard to the agents used, fig. 9 warrants the conclusion that the importance of barbiturates has significantly diminished in three successive five-year periods. Yet representatives of this group continue taking the lion's share of drugs used in self-intoxication. A striking feature of this

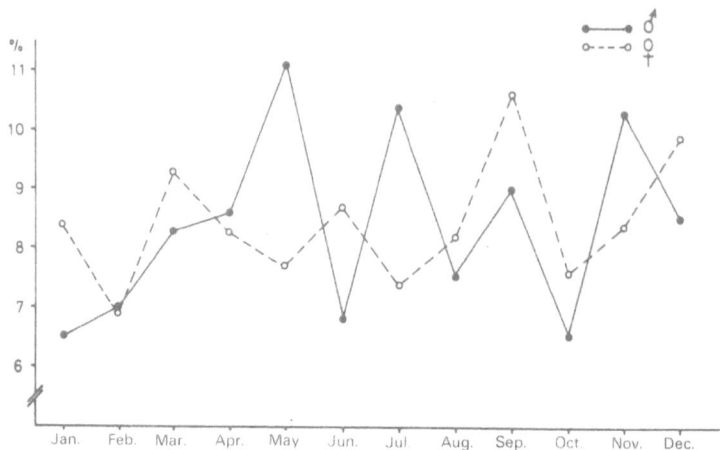

Figure 8. Monthly percentages of total self-intoxication admissions.

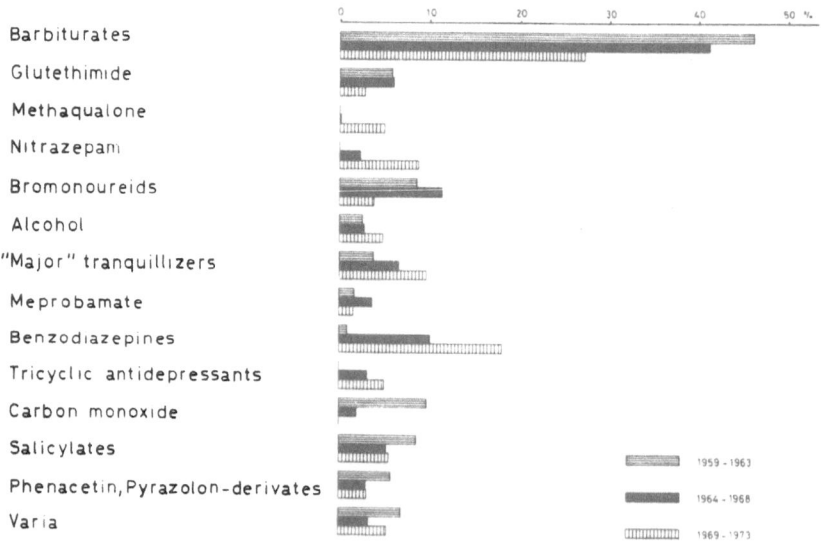

Figure 9. Agents used for self-poisoning in three successive five-year periods. "Major" tranquillizers were mainly phenothiazine derivatives.

pattern is increased use of nitrazepam and other benzodiazepines. Intentional carbon monoxide poisoning has not been observed in our department since 1968, when natural gas was introduced in Amsterdam. Another conspicuous feature in the rapidly increasing tendency to take several drugs simultaneously (fig. 10); this, too, corroborates international experience. Fig. 11 shows the duration of coma as a cumulative plot. Nearly 60 percent

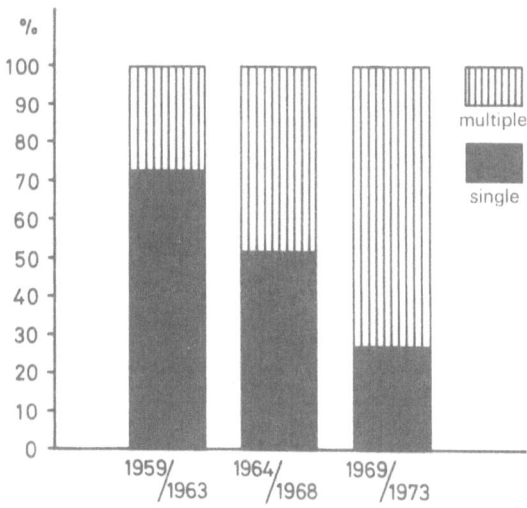

Figure 10. Percentages of single-drug and multiple-drug intoxications.

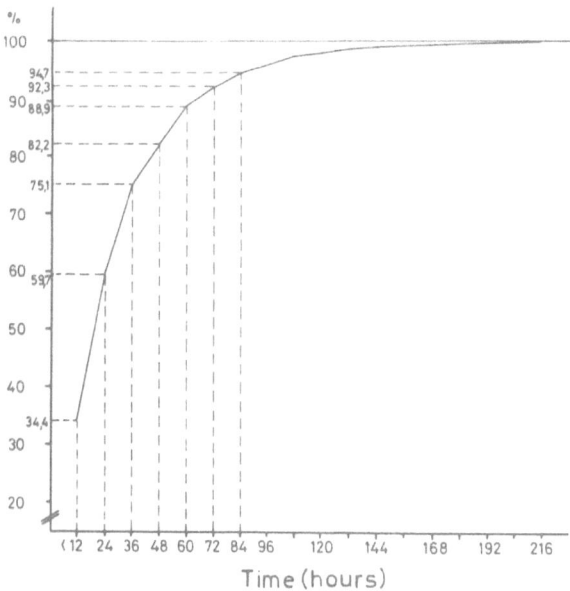

Figure 11. Duration of coma.

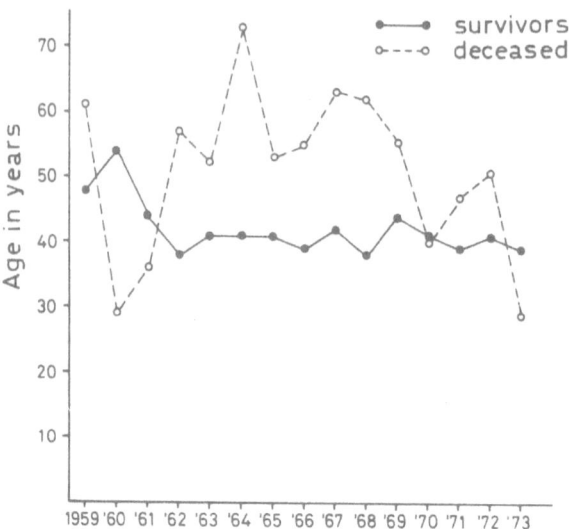

Figure 12. Mean ages of survivors and deceased in each year.

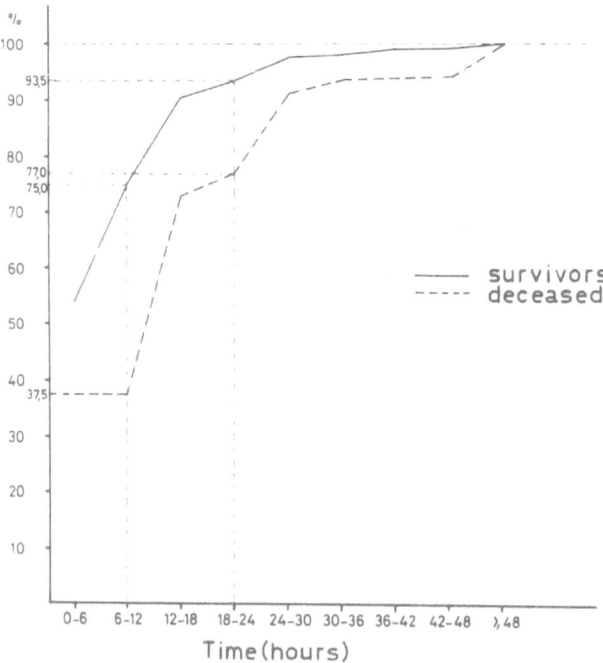

Figure 13. Interval between ingestion of drugs and arrival at hospital, for survivors and deceased, cumulatively recorded.

of our patients regained consciousness within 24 hours, this group including a number of patients who were not comatose at all. Slightly over 80 percent of patients regained consciousness within 48 hours.

All patients were seen by a psychiatrist before discharge. On his advice, one third of all patients were transferred to a mental hospital after recovery; two thirds were allowed to return home.

Finally, I should like to mention that our epidemiological study permits two conclusions which proved to have prognostic importance. First, fig. 12 shows that the prognosis for older patients was worse than that for the younger ones. The deceased had a higher average age than those who recovered, the difference being statistically significant. Secondly, the cumulative plot in fig. 13 clearly shows that patients in the group of fatal cases had on the average a significantly longer interval between the ingestion of drugs and hospital admission than those who survived their self-intoxication. This difference, too, was significant.

With few exceptions, all patients received conservative supportive therapy. In view of the two above mentioned findings the question arises whether it might not be advisable to take measures ensuring accelerated elimination of the drug taken in high-risk patients.

CONCLUSIONS

A survey is presented of the cases of self-intoxication admitted to the Department of Internal Medicine, Amsterdam University Hospital, over a fifteen-year period from 1959 to 1974, when these patients accounted for about 10 percent of all admissions to the abovementioned department. The number of female patients always exceeded that of male patients. Most patients were found to be in age group 20–30. There was no demonstrable seasonal in influence on the rate of admission for self-intoxication. Barbiturates were the agents most frequently used for self-intoxication, although the relative frequency was decreasing over the years. There is an increasing tendency to take several drugs simultaneously. Some 60 percent of all patients had regained consciousness after 24 hours, and 80 percent after 48 hours. One third of all patients had to be transferred to a mental hospital. It was found that the prognosis was less good when the patients had been left untreated longer, and when they belonged to older age groups.

REFERENCES

Baker, A.B., Early treatment of the unconscious patient suffering from drug overdose. *Med. J. Australia* 1, 497—503 (1969) .
Matthew, H. and Lawson, A.A.H., Acute barbiturate poisoning, a review of two years experience. *Quart. J. Med.* 35, 539–552 (1966).

Smith, A.J., Self-poisoning with drugs: a worsening situation. *Brit. Med. J.* 4, 157–160 (1972).

Timmers, H., 15-jaar zelfvergiftigingen in de interne kliniek." Thesis, Amsterdam, 1975.

16. LABORATORY DIAGNOSIS OF INTOXICATIONS

B. WIDDOP

Although the incidence of poisoning continues to rise in many countries, the overall mortality for this condition in hospitals remains low (table 1). Nevertheless, the work load placed on hospital services is considerable and, in some areas can constitute almost ten percent of all emergency medical admissions. In modern society, drugs, in particular those with psychotropic activity, are by far the commonest agents involved (table 2). Fortunately, the majority of patients respond to the widely adopted procedures of supportive treatment and laboratory aid consists mainly of biochemical measurements (blood gases, electrolytes, enzymes) which gauge the physiological status of the patient. Some clinicians who are familiar with drug intoxication, especially those who are attached to Poisons Treatment centres, claim that, in general, any accurate chemical identification of the drug ingested has no bearing on the management of the patient. Clinical toxicologists are far from ubiquitous, however, and where patients are admitted to emergency reception centres they will most likely be dealt

Table 1. Yearly admissions and mortality of poisoned patients in hospital (England and Wales 1956–1972).

Year	1956	1961	1963	1965	1967	1972
Admissions	23,300	27,900	45,900	53,000	67,300	105,000
Deaths	445	541	887	888	801	736
Mortality (%)	1.9	1.9	1.9	1.6	1.2	0.7

Table 2. Analysis of enquiries received by the National Poisons Information Service (London) during 1975.

Type of poison	Number of enquiries
Drugs	10,972
Household chemicals and cosmetic agents	5,795
Plants	1,572
Agricultural chemicals	1,342
Industrial chemicals	573
Miscellaneous	647
Total	20,901

with by physicians less confident that the cause of the patient's illness is poisoning and not some other organic disorder. Relatives and friends can prove the most unreliable sources of circumstantial evidence and drugs and medicines found in the vicinity of the unconscious patient, although useful clues in a preliminary toxicological search, may have played no part in the episode whatsoever. Drug intoxications are further complicated by the propensity of those who embark on such a course to ingest a variety of agents simultaneously (table 3). The subsequent clinical features arising from this exercise in polypharmacy may confuse, if not completely mislead, even the most experienced physicians. In such circumstances, a laboratory capable of furnishing rapid qualitative data can be invaluable.

The need to perform quantitative assays is more difficult to justify except in those cases where the nature of the toxin and the quantity taken may warrant active therapy such as the administration of antidotes, which may increase the distress of the patient, or the application of elimination proceddures (forced diuresis, haemodialysis, haemoperfusion) which place an additional burden on the physician's skills and time. The decision to invoke or withold such measures can often hinge on measuring the circulating levels of the toxic agent.

The practice of chemical toxicology has, in the past, been largely confined to departments of forensic medicine or clinical chemistry. Recent years have seen the establishment of toxicological laboratories operating in their own right on a regional or supra-regional basis. This contribution is based on experience gained in one of these laboratories, the Poisons Unit at Guy's Hospital in London. It aims to describe some of the analytical problems encountered, how the service is organized and, finally, highlights those incidents for which these endeavours are most appropriate.

Table 3. Medication prescribed for a female patient admitted unconscious after multiple overdosage.

Medication	Overdosage
Tryptizol	Amitriptyline*
Surmontil	Trimipramine*
Niamid	Nialamide*
Librium	Chlordiazepoxide*
Optimax	L-Tryptophan
	Pyridoxine
	Ascorbic acid
Hexopal	Inositol
Feospan	Ferrous Sulphate

* Detected in urine and plasma.

COMMUNICATION WITH THE LABORATORY

It is undeniable that a large proportion of requests for toxicological investigations which impinge on a busy laboratory are initially viewed with suspicion by those called upon to perform the analyses. Few clinicians are versed at a practical level in the difficulties involved in meeting their demands. Far fewer in number are the laboratory workers who are able to comprehend the anxieties faced by those who are charged with the welfare of a poisoned patient. The mediator between the two groups should be a clinician who has sound knowledge of the pharmacology and toxicology of drugs together with personal experience in the management of intoxicated patients. He should be responsible for filtering through to the laboratory those requests for which there is a valid reason for analysis and, conversely, rejecting requests which may reassure the clinician but have little or no relevance to patient management. Where the analyses are thought to be of value, the mediator can instruct the clinician as regards the appropriate samples to be collected and, following completion of the analyses, give an informed interpretation of the findings. In the specialist laboratory, such a role, which is most adequately filled by a clinical pharmacologist, is of paramount importance.

COLLECTION OF SAMPLES

The type of sample and the appropriate volume is governed by the analytical procedure in use and varies between laboratories. Any specific requirements should be ascertained when first making contact with the laboratory. In general, however, samples of gastric contents, blood, and/or urine will suffice for most overdose investigations.

Gastric contents
Vomit, gastric aspirate or gastric lavage are the most useful samples for qualitative analyses. If obtained shortly after ingestion of the overdose they may contain recognizable tablets or capsules. In addition, they may emit characteristic odours (e.g. methyl salicylate, paraldehyde, phenelzine, ethchlorvynol) which yield immediate clues to analysts with a trained olfactory faculty. Further bonuses are the absence of degradation products (metabolites) which complicate certain assays and the fact that the drugs are present in abundance. These samples are of little use, however, if a considerable length of time has elapsed after ingestion since the toxin may then have passed from the stomach into the small intestine. By the same token, the clinician should be careful to collect and despatch

the first portion of the gastric lavage for analysis and not subsequent fractions which, following successful treatment, may be devoid of the toxic agent.

Urine

Most conscious patients will readily void a urine specimen but in the comatose patient, catheterization is necessary. Whether this is justifiable in all cases, in view of the reputedly high incidence of urinary tract infection subsequent to this procedure, is debatable. Nevertheless, from an analytical viewpoint, this fluid is invaluable. It becomes essential when drugs have been self-administered by the intravenous route and especially when, even following overdosage, these drugs appear in the blood in concentrations which defy detection by all but the most refined analytical techniques. The presence of drug metabolites in urine can be a hindrance to identification or, alternatively, a blessing, particularly when chromatographic techniques which can simultaneously characterize the parent drug and its degradation products are applied. For a comprehensive qualitative drug screen, approximately 50 ml of urine should be collected on admission of the patient and preferably before the administration of any drugs to treat the overdose syndrome. Should this already have occurred, the clinician is beholden to inform the laboratory since these agents may interfere with the analytical tests. The use of preservatives should be avoided since, again, their presence can mislead the analyst.

Blood

When the cause of the intoxication is completely unknown, blood should never be regarded as the sample of choice for qualitative screening. Modern drugs such as tricyclic antidepressants, phenothiazines, opiate derivatives and benzodiazepines have a tendency to be sequestered in the tissues at the expense of the blood with the result that the amounts available for detection are extremely low. This sample is preferably reserved for any quantitative exercises which become necessary subsequent to the preliminary testing of gastric contents or urine. Few measurements are carried out on whole blood, the analyst preferring to work with the purer matrix of serum or plasma. The sample should be withdrawn and dispensed with care. For example, the vigorous discharge of blood via a syringe needle will flood the serum with haemoglobin and completely invalidate a serum iron assay. Where ethyl alcohol ingestion is clinically obvious, blood for alcohol assay should be dispensed into tubes containing sodium fluoride to guard against changes in the alcohol content brought about by extraneous organisms. It is not unknown for analysts to receive blood samples for lithium assay dispensed into lithium-heparin tubes! As emphasized previously, advice on the exact requirements is readily available from the laboratory concerned. A 10 ml sample of whole blood or, alternatively 5 ml of plasma or serum, is adequate for most purposes.

The above recommendations apply to ideal situations and where infants or patients with renal failure are involved, the clinician may be unable to comply with these. Experienced analysts can generally be prevailed upon to modify their requirements, however, provided such mitigating circumstances are made known and useful information can foreseeably be gained from the samples which are available.

Finally, it is mandatory that the specimens be clearly labelled with the patient's full name, hospital ward and, without fail, the date and time of collection. The clinician should personally ensure that the appropriate means of transporting the specimens to the laboratory is secured without delay.

METHODS FOR DRUG DETECTION AND MEASUREMENT

The so-called "spot-tests" are extremely simple, require the minimum of expertise and can be applied to small samples (1 ml) of either gastric contents or urine. Thus, by the addition of reagents which elicit characteristic colours, the analyst can readily discern the presence of iron, salicylates, paracetamol, phenothiazines, imipramine, chloral hydrate and dichloral-phenazone (Meade et al. 1972). For other drugs, some form of purification away from the endogenous constituents of the sample matrix is necessary and the most widely adopted procedure is that of solvent extraction. A typical scheme is that devised by Berry and Grove (1973) whereby urine or gastric contents (10 ml) are acidified and extracted with an equivalent volume of chloroform to retrieve acidic and neutral drugs such as the barbiturates, glutethimide and methaqualone. A further aliquot of the specimen is made alkaline and extracted with 10 ml of diethyl ether. This takes out the chemically basic drugs which include phenothiazines, tricyclic antidepressants, opiates and amphetamines. After centrifugation to separate the aqueous and organic layers, these latter are removed and evaporated to a small volume. This procedure yields relatively pure and concentrated organic solutions of the drugs which are then amenable to chemical and physicochemical investigation. The nature and intensity of these is largely dependent on the time and equipment available to the analyst. In the past, much reliance was placed on determining the ultra-violet absorption characteristics of sample extracts (Sunshine and Gerber 1963). This technique, though not without its merits, is inapplicable in cases of multiple overdose where the resultant spectrum may be a composite of several drugs and their metabolites. Needless to say, it is totally un-rewarding when drugs with an insignificant or nonexistent capacity to absorb ultra-violet radiation have been ingested. In recent years, analytical toxicologists have favoured techniques which resolve (or chromatograph) the components of sample extracts prior to their detection by chemical or physical means. In its simplest form this involves applying several aliquotes of the sample extract to one end of a silica-coated sheet of glass or plastic which is then placed vertically in a tank containing a mixture of solvents. This mixture travels symmetrically across the silica layer, carrying in its wake any drugs and metabolites present in the extract. These are mobilized at different rates according to their chemical structures such that on removing the plate from the developing tank they are deposited in discrete regions as compact spots. Their detection and identification rests on their position relative to simultaneously chromatographed authentic drugs and their behaviour towards a sequence of colourimetric reagents sprayed onto the plate (Zingales 1967, 1968; Berry and Grove 1973). This versatile and inexpensive technique of thin-layer chromatography is ideally suited for use in non-specialized clinical chemistry laboratories.

In the well-endowed laboratory, all manner of refined instrumentation can be brought to bear in qualitative exercises. Thus, the literature is replete with schemes invoking gas-liquid chromatography (GC) (Finkle et al. 1971; Proelss and Lohmann 1971; Rice and Wilson 1973; Griffiths and Diamond 1974). High-pressure liquid chromatography (HPLC), with its unlimited potential to separate and detect both lipid soluble and polar (non-extractable) drugs and their metabolites, is rapidly emerging as a screening device (Chan et al. 1974). Mass-spectrometry (MS), a technique which, in a sense, furnishes a spectral fingerprint of the drug, is now used routinely in some centres (Law et al. 1972; Billets et al. 1973; Boerner et al. 1973). Hybrid computerized instruments (GC-MS) are even more powerful tools, though prohibitively expensive (Hammar et al. 1969; Finkle et al. 1972) .

On an emergency basis, only salicylates, paracetamol, iron, lithium, barbiturates, alcohols, glutethimide, methaqualone, meprobamate and ethchlorvynol need be measured in blood or serum. The first three agents are among the few which are readily determined in overdose concentrations. The barbiturates and related hypnotics present more of a problem. Colourimetric and spectroscopic methods for this group are fraught with interference from other drugs, endogenous blood constituents and laboratory contaminants (Tompsett 1969). In addition, they fail to differentiate between long-acting varieties (e.g. phenobarbitone) and the intermediate-acting congeners. Again, chromatographic procedures, especially gas-liquid chromatography, are the methods of choice (Leach and Toseland 1968; Flanagan and Berry 1977). The measurement of other drugs in blood is of little relevance in directing treatment, but does serve to confirm that a drug detected by the initial qualitative screen is present to a toxic degree.

INTERPRETATION OF FINDINGS

Despite a thoroughgoing scrutiny of the urine or gastric contents, the findings are never categorical. If negative results have been achieved, this may immediately lead the clinician to consider an alternative diagnosis to poisoning. Less likely, though not unknown, is the possibility that the gastric aspirate has been recovered after the stomach has emptied its contents into the duodenum. Conversely, a urine specimen may have been voided prior to the accumulation of a detectable concentration in the bladder. This emphasizes the desirability of collecting both types of samples for analysis. Finally, it should never be assumed that any analytical scheme of drug detection is totally comprehensive.

Positive findings are, paradoxically, more difficult to interpret. Even the simplest tests may be sufficiently sensitive to detect therapeutic concentration of drugs. Thus, a patient may have taken these quite legitimately and be suffering from an organic disorder. Alternatively, an inexperienced analyst may have discontinued his search at the first sign of a positive result and, in so doing, failed to detect the true causative agent. For example, a male patient was admitted unconscious and smelling of alcohol. The clinical chemistry laboratory confirmed the presence of alcohol by a urine test, but the patient deteriorated and died 24 hours later. Forensic analysis of the original specimens disclosed a blood alcohol level of minimum import (1.1 g/l) together with a highly toxic salicylate level of 1200 ng/l. It is reasonable to presume that with prompt alkaline diuresis, this patient would have survived. Equally pressing is the need to exclude a biochemical lesion without delay. Thus, a Swedish visitor to London was discovered unconscious in his hotel room. Poisoning was suspected and the patient was admitted to a London teaching hospital and treated supportively for several hours. Meanwhile, a distant toxicology laboratory screened samples of his urine for drugs. A thorough search revealed an insignificant amount of a biguanide antidiabetic agent. A urine "clinistix" test was strongly positive for glucose, but by the time this information was relayed to the ward the uncontrolled diabetic was dead.

Table 4 is included as a guide to the interpretation of blood drug level measurements. These tenets are by no means universal, however, and in considering the question, "Do the quantitative findings correlate with the condition of the patient?", each case must be considered on its merits. Individuals vary enormously in their tolerance to a toxic insult according to their previous exposure to drugs and their physical health. Multiple

Table 4. Interpretation of toxicological data: drug concentrations (mg/l).

Drug	Therapeutic levels: less than	Levels associated with severe toxicity
Alcohols		
Ethanol	–	300
Methanol	–	200
Barbiturates		
Barbitone	15	100
Phenobarbitone	30	100
Others	5	50
Benzodiazepines		
Diazepam (Valium)	1.0	5.0
Nitrazepam (Mogadon)	0.2	2.0
Ethchlorvynol	20	100
Glutethimide	4	40
Meprobamate	20	40
Methaqualone	4	20
Paracetamol	20	200–300[a] 100–150[b]
Salicylate	250	600
Trichloroethanol[c]	20	100
Tricyclic antidepressants		
Amitriptyline and metabolite (nortriptyline)	0.18	1.0
Nortriptyline	0.15	1.0

a. Four hours after ingestion.
b. Twelve hours after ingestion.
c. Major metabolite of chloral hydrate and dichloralphenazone.

overdosage may produce synergism where the combined effect of two drugs is more pronounced than that normally elicited by the independent activity of each drug. The popular "cocktail" of alcohol and barbiturates is a common example of this phenomenon.

A further question, often posed, is "How will the patient fare subsequently?" Tentative predictions, based on the supposition that the pharmacological effects of a drug subside in parallel with its decline in the blood, can be made from half-life data. Much of these data derive from single low-dose studies in healthy volunteers and should not be extrapolated to overdose situations too rigidly. Many hours may elapse before a massive quantity of drug is completely absorbed. Collins (1970) encountered a case of Carbrital (pentobarbitone and carbromal) poisoning where the blood concentrations of both drugs rose continually for 50 hours after ingestion (fig. 1). The accuracy of these predictions is further mitigated where drugs with anticholinergic activity (e.g. opiates, tricyclic antidepressants) inhibit both their own absorption and that of concurrently ingested drugs (Widdop 1974).

Even when absorption is complete, it cannot be assumed that the processes of metabolism and excretion will function according to normal patterns.

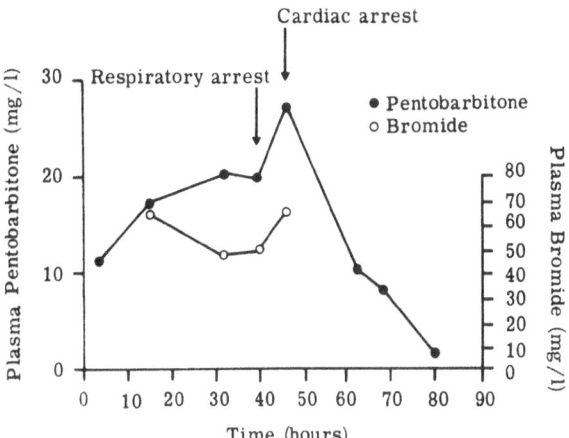

Figure 1. Plasma concentration of pentobarbitone and total bromide in a case of Carbrital overdose (Collins 1970).

Grove and Toseland (1971) demonstrated a clear inhibition of the liver detoxification capacities of patients severely poisoned with amylobarbitone. Conversely, a liver which has been activated by chronic drug exposure may be more susceptible to damage by agents which are metabolized to toxic products. Prescott et al. (1971) suggested that patients who took barbiturates or were chronic alcoholics might be less tolerant to the hepatotoxic effects of paracetamol.

Finally, renal impairment will modify excretion patterns, but its significance is limited to those drugs for which this is a major route of elimination (e.g. salicylates, barbitone, phenobarbitone, digoxin).

APPLICATIONS OF TOXICOLOGICAL ANALYSES

Brief mention has already been made of some of the applications of drug analyses and this warrants further expansion.

Differential diagnosis of poisoning or organic disorder
This aspect is best illustrated by reference to a typical incident dealt with by the Poisons Unit laboratory. This concerned a young man with no previous history of abnormalities who collapsed shortly after entering a public house. On admission to hospital he was deeply unconscious and required mechanical ventilation. Lumbar puncture yielded blood-stained cerebrospinal fluid. but arteriograms showed no abnormalities. A toxicological screen suggested overdosage with amitriptyline, paracetamol,

dextropropoxyphene and chlordiazepoxide. A repeat lumbar puncture gave clear CSF and the patient recovered uneventfully after supportive therapy.

Diagnosis of brain death
Following a conference of the Medical Royal Colleges and their Faculties in 1976, a statement was issued setting out diagnostic criteria for brain death (*British Medical Journal* 1976). Among the recommendations were that depressant drugs with prolonged durations of action should be excluded as a cause of deep coma. This was thought to be particularly important in patients whose primary cause of coma lay in the toxic effects of drugs followed by anoxic cerebral damage. Equally, it was felt that persistent effects of hypnotics and narcotics should be excluded as a cause of respiratory failure. The role of the toxicology laboratory in this realm is self-evident.

Detection of non-accidental poisoning in children
The abuse of children by parents or guardians is not limited to physical violence or nutritional and emotional neglect. Assault by administration of drugs probably occurs more frequently than is realized (Weston et al. 1968). The Guy's Hospital Poisons Unit has recently assisted the clinicians of a major London paediatric hospital in disclosing six cases of non-accidental child poisoning which fell into this category (Rogers et al. 1976) and thirteen subsequent cases, as yet unpublished, have been encountered. Notwithstanding their crucial role in rapidly confirming the diagnosis, toxicological analyses provide substantial evidence when legal protection is sought for the child.

Monitoring of drug abuse
Toxicological laboratories can render a considerable service to psychiatrists who specialize in the control and treatment of drug dependence. Techniques analogous to those previously cited for overdose screening (Berry and Grove 1971) can be applied to the routine screening of addicts' urines for the presence of opiates, amphetamines, phenothiazines, barbiturates and other hypnotics. In this way the psychiatrist is guarded against the unwarranted prescribing of dangerous drugs to pseudo-addicts and can monitor his progress in treating the genuine dependent. The early detection of changing trends in drug abuse is an additional benefit. Incidents where psychiatrists call for laboratory aid in differentiating endogenous mental illness from mental aberrations induced by psychotomimetic agents (e.g. cannabis, LSD) occur frequently.

Influence on active therapy of drug overdosage
The treatment of iron salts or paracetamol overdosage by the parenteral

administration of antidotes with their own intrinsic toxicity (i.e. desfer-rioxamine and cysteamine respectively) is more rational when the clinician is armed with analytical evidence for the degree of intoxication. Indeed, for paracetamol poisoning, where the early clinical features can be mis-leadingly mild, a blood paracetamol estimation may be vital in prompting antidotal therapy in time to prevent the onset of hepatic lesions (Gazzard et al. 1977).

The elimination techniques of forced diuresis, peritoneal dialysis and haemodialysis are effective only with regard to poisoning with salicylates, barbitone, phenobarbitone and alcohols. Haemoperfusion has wider appli-cations in that it will also remove intermediate-acting barbiturates, methaqualone, chloral hydrate, meprobamate and ethchlorvynol – see table 5 (Vale et al. 1975; Widdop et al. 1975). Nevertheless, these measures are totally futile when drugs with large distribution volumes have been ingested (Crome et al. 1978; Iversen et al. 1978). Physicians intending to institute these procedures should obtain preliminary analytical confirmation that a drug has been taken which is amenable to removal and that its concentration in the blood is high enough to guarantee a substantial re-duction in the body load – see table 6 (Volans et al. 1977).

CONCLUSION

Sufficient evidence has, hopefully, been presented here to justify the existence of well-equipped laboratories staffed by chemists and bio-

Table 5. Applications of elimination procedures to drug removal in the intoxicated patient.

Elimination technique	Drugs removed in significant amounts
Forced diuresis	Alcohols
	Barbitone
	Phenobarbitone
	Salicylates
Haemodialysis	Alcohols
	Barbitone
	Phenobarbitone
	Lithium
Charcoal haemoperfusion	All barbiturates
	Carbromal
	Glutethimide
	Ethchlorvynol
	Meprobamate
	Methaqualone
	Trichloroethanol
	Salicylates

Table 6. Plasma drug level criteria used in selecting patients for haemoper-
        fusion therapy.

Drug	Plasma concentration (mg/l)
Phenobarbitone and barbitone	100
Other barbiturates	50
Glutethimide	40
Methaqualone	40
Ethchlorvynol	100
Meprobamate	100
Trichloroethanol	50
Salicylates	800

chemists offering a regional toxicological service. Clearly, these will
function most efficiently where the population density is high. Rapid
transport of samples via road and rail is accomplished with ease in urban
areas. For outlying hospitals, however, especially in those countries with
underdeveloped transport systems, the difficulties involved in conveying
specimens to the laboratory within a reasonable period of time may be
insurmountable. Bach and Dennis (1977) recently highlighted this problem
with respect to South Africa and drew attention to the need to supply
clinicians working in rural areas with simple diagnostic aids. Admittedly,
Phenistix (Curry 1976) will detect salicylates, para-aminosalicylate,
chlorpromazine and tetracyclines. The Merckoquant dipstick will react
with ferrous iron in gastric aspirate and a semi-quantitative test kit for
blood paracetamol measurement is now available (Kendal et al. 1976).
Much remains to be done in this direction, however, and it may be that
the burgeoning development of immunological assay kits will serve to fill
this gap (Sunshine 1974).

REFERENCES

Bach, P.H. and Dennis, M., Diagnosis of acute poisoning. S.A. Med. J. 51, 958 (1977).
Berry, D.J. and Grove, J., Improved chromatographic techniques and their interpretation
    for the screening of urine from drug-dependent subjects. J. Chromatogr. 61, 111 (1971).
Berry, D.J. and Grove, J., Emergency toxicological screening for drugs commonly taken in
    overdose. J. Chromatogr. 80, 205 (1973).
Billets, S., Carruth, J., Einolf, N., Ward, R. and Fenselan, C., Rapid identification of acute
    drug intoxications. Hopkins Med. J. 133, 148 (1973).
Boerner, U., Abbott, S., Eidson, J.C., Becker, C.E., Horio, T. and Loeffler, K., Direct
    mass-spectrometric analysis of body fluids from acutely poisoned patients. Clin.
    Chim. Acta 49, 445 (1973).
British Medical Journal, Diagnosis of brain death. Br. Med. J. 2, 1187 (1976).
Chan, M.L., Whetsell, C. and McChesney, J.D., Use of high-pressure liquid chromatography
    for the separation of drugs of abuse. J. Chromatogr. Sci. 12, 512 (1974).
Collins, J., A case of self-poisoning with carbrital. Postgrad. Med. J. 46, 584 (1970).

Crome, P., Hampel, G., Vale, J.A., Volans, G.N., Widdop, B. and Goulding, R., Haemo-perfusion in treatment of drug intoxication. *Brit. Med. J.* 1, 174 (1978).

Curry, A.S., *Poisons Detection in Human Organs*, 3rd ed., Springfield, 1976, p. 66.

Finkle, B.S., Cherry, E.J. and Taylor, D.M., A GLC based system for the detection of poisons drugs and human metabolites encountered in forensic toxicology. *J. Chromatogr. Sci.* 9, 393 (1971).

Finkle, B.S., Taylor, M. and Bonelli, E., A GC/MS reference data system for the identification of drugs of abuse. *J. Chromatogr. Sci.* 10, 312 (1972).

Flanagan, R.J. and Berry, D.J., Routine analysis of barbiturates and some other hypnotics in the blood plasma as an aid to the diagnosis of acute poisoning. *J. Chromatogr.* 131, 131 (1977).

Gazzard, B.G., Hughes, R.D., Widdop, B., Goulding, R., Davis, M. and Williams, R., Early prediction of the outcome of a paracetamol overdose based on an analysis of 163 patients. *Postgrad. Med. J.* 53, 243 (1977).

Griffiths, W.C. and Diamond, I., Emergency testing and routine monitoring of therapeutic drugs in a comprehensive analytical system. *Clin. Toxicol.* 7, 365 (1974).

Grove, J. and Toseland, P.A., Excretion of hydroxyamylobarbitone in man: the importance of the hydroxyamylobarbitone/amylobarbitone ratio. *Ann. Clin. Biochem.* 8, 109 (1971).

Hammar, C.G., Holmstredt, B., Lindgren, J.E. and Tham, R., The combination of gas-chromatography and mass-spectrometry in the identification of drugs and metabolites. *Adv. Pharmacol. Chemother.* 7, 53 (1969).

Iversen, B.M., Willassen, Y. and Bakke, O.M., Charcoal haemoperfusion in nortriptyline poisoning. *Lancet* 1, 388 (1978).

Kendal, S., Lloyd-Jones, G. and Smith, C.F., The development of a blood paracetamol estimation kit. *J. Int. Med. Res.* 4, Suppl. 4, 83 (1976).

Law, N.C., Fales, H.M. and Milne, G.W.A., Identification of drugs taken in overdose cases. *Clin. Toxicol.* 5, 17 (1972).

Leach, H. and Toseland, P.A., The determination of barbiturates and some related drugs by gas-chromatography. *Clin. Chim. Acta* 20, 195 (1968).

Meade, B.W., Widdop, B., Blackmore, D.J., Brown, S.S., Curry, A.S., Goulding, R., Higgins, G., Matthew, H.J.S. and Rinsler, M.G., Simple tests to detect poisons. *Ann. Clin. Biochem.* 9, 35 (1972).

Prescott, L.F., Wright, N., Roscoe, P. and Brown, S.S., Plasma paracetamol half-life and hepatic necrosis in patients with paracetamol overdosage. *Lancet* 1, 519 (1971).

Proelss, H.F. and Lohmann, H.J., Profile of sedatives and tranquillizers in serum, as measured by gas-liquid chromatography. *Clin. Chem.* 17, 222 (1971).

Rice, A.J. and Wilson, W.R., 'Rapid identification of drugs in body fluids of comatose patients. *Clin Toxicol.* 6, 59 (1973).

Rogers, D., Tripp, J., Bentovim, A., Robinson, A., Berry, D. and Goulding, R., Non-accidental poisoning: an extended syndrome of child abuse. *Br. Med. J.* 1, 793 (1976).

Sunshine, I., Immunoassay of drugs. In: *The Poisoned Patient: The Role of the Laboratory.* Ed., Porter, R. and O'Connor, M., Amsterdam, 1974.

Sunshine, I. and Gerber, S.R., *Spectrophotometric Analysis of Drugs Including Atlas of Spectra.* Springfield, 1963.

Tompsett, S.L., Interference from the presence of other substances in detecting and determin-ing barbiturates in biological material. *J. Clin. Pathol.* 22, 291 (1969).

Vale, A.J., Rees, A.J., Widdop, B. and Goulding, R., Use of charcoal haemoperfusion in the management of severely poisoned patients. *Br. Med. J.* 1, 5 (1975).

Volans, G.N., Vale, J.A., Crome, P., Widdop, B. and Goulding, R., The role of charcoal haemoperfusion in the management of acute poisoning by drugs. In: *Artificial Organs: Proceedings of a Seminar on the Clinical Applications of Membrane Oxygenation and Sorbent-Based Systems.* Ed., Kenedi, R.M., et al., London, 1977.

Weston, J.T., Helfer, R.E. and Kempe, C.H. (eds.), *Battered Child*, Chicago, 1968.

Widdop, B., Drug analysis in the overdosed patient. In: *The Poisoned Patient: The Role of the Laboratory.* Ed., Porter, R. and O'Connor, M., Amsterdam, 1974.

Widdop, B., Medd, R.K., Braithwaite, R.A., Rees, A.J. and Goulding, R., Experimental drug intoxication: Treatment with charcoal haemoperfusion *Arch. Toxicol.*, 34, 27 (1975).

Zingales, I., Systematic identification of psychotropic drugs by thin-layer chromatography I. *J. Chromatogr.* 31, 405 (1967).

Zingales, I., Systematic identification of psychotropic drugs by thin-layer chromatography II. *J. Chromatogr.* 34, 44 (1968).

17. THE ROLE OF THE LABORATORY IN THE TREATMENT OF INTOXICATIONS WITH DRUGS

A.N.P. VAN HEIJST

The treatment of an intoxicated patient has changed in the course of time. Hippocrates claimed that for every poison an antidote was available, a statement which held out for a very long time. In the English Pharmacopoeia in 1746 an antidote consisting of 46 components was described. Indicated as an antidote were products with an action opposite to the pharmacological action of the poison. Even today many physicians asking for information at the National Poisons Information Centre are really surprised when they are told that the number of antidotes useful for cases of acute intoxications can be counted on the fingers of one hand, since the supply of all the different antidotes to the patient was often a disaster. Perhaps as an antidote against the complex of antidotes still used, the so-called "Scandinavian method" of therapy, based on refusing every active interference with the poison, was introduced in 1963. The maintainance of the vital functions of the organism, such as respiration and circulation, was the principle task. The success of this treatment by these "nihilists", as they were called, was evident; mortality decreased from 25 percent to less than 1 percent.

Many of the clinical toxicologists were satisfied; others on the contrary refused to accept the long duration of the coma, which could persist for four to five days in serious intoxications with hypnotics. Complications such as respiratory infections and circulatory insufficiency increased mortality, so more emphasis was laid on an increase in elimination of the toxic product. The first step was the introduction of forced diuresis. Administration of about one litre of fluid per hour intravenously to obtain a urine production of one litre per hour, with the aid of diuretics, provided to be effective. The combination of forced diuresis with alkalinization in phenobarbital, barbital and salicylate intoxications or acidification in severe amphetamine and quinine intoxications resulted in a considerably higher clearance. A great disadvantage was the load on the circulation which was a great risk in patients with hypotension. The use of haemodialysis to eliminate toxic drugs from the plasma was advocated, and it proved to be more successful than forced diuresis. Nevertheless haemodialysis was only seldom applied, an important reason was that it could be applied only in intoxications with hydrophilic drugs.

In the last few years haemoperfusion has been available. In an extracorporeal system the blood is conducted over coated charcoal or resin. With this system, the clearance of the poison from the circulation is very high. The difference in clearance between forced diuresis and haemoperfusion can be shown in the elimination rate of barbital (fig. 1) and cyclobarbital (fig. 2) in a combined intoxication in a 68-year old female. By applying two perfusions of three and four hours respectively with an interval of twelve hours, an amount of 4.4 g barbital and 1.4 g cyclobarbital was eliminated while a forced diuresis took 36 hours to eliminate 2.2 g barbital and 0.53 g cyclobarbital (de Groot et al. 1977). With the introduction of more aggressive methods such as haemodialysis and haemoperfusion the question arises which are the decisive criteria to be taken into account for use of these

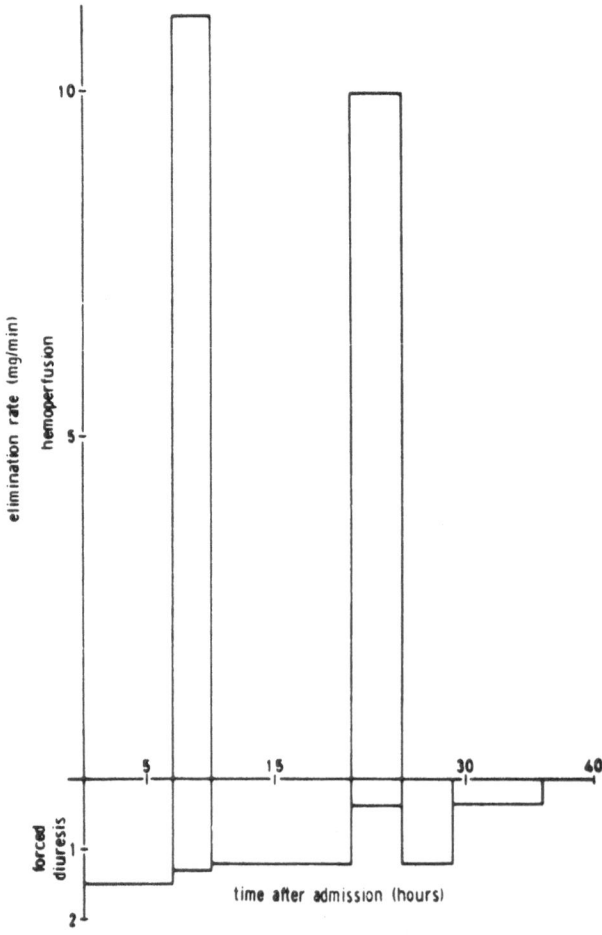

Figure 1. Barbital elimination rates in a patient with a combined intoxication of barbital and cyclobarbital; comparison of haemoperfusion and forced diuresis.

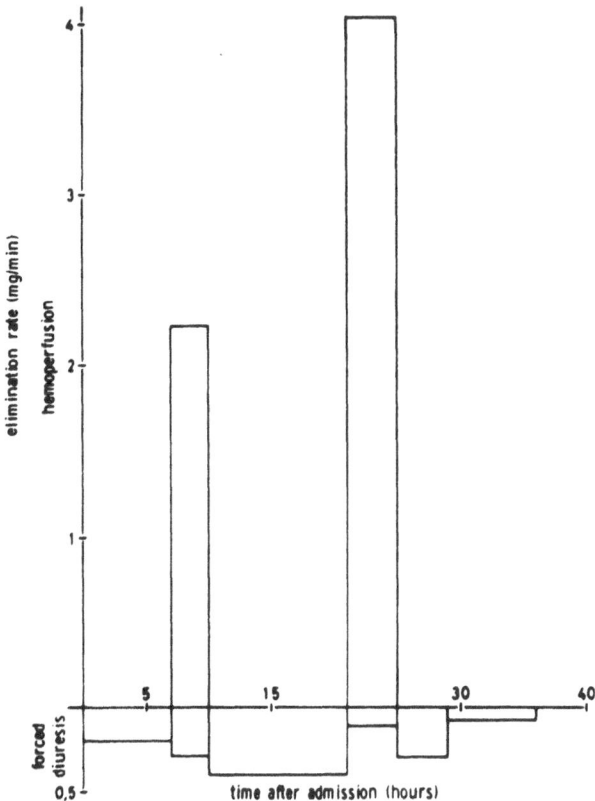

Figure 2. Cyclobarbital elimination rates in the same patient.

techniques. To know these criteria is necessary because these techniques are not without risk for the patient. For instance, large blood vessels must be cannulated; blood clotting is diminished; there is a fall in the number of leucocytes and a substantial decrease in the number of thrombocytes. Another reason for the establishment of strict indications of these procedures is an economic one. The apparatus and the specialized staff are very expensive. In our opinion haemodialysis and haemoperfusion can only be justified if performed by staff daily occupied with these techniques. The first criterium in intoxications with hypnotics and sedatives is the clinical condition of the patient: the patient must be in deep coma without reactions to pain, and all reflexes being absent. The second criterium is a high plasma level.

Since 1975 a research programme in collaboration with the Laboratory of Analytical Toxicology (Prof. Dr. R.A.A. Maes) has been set up to obtain a better insight into the correlation between clinical symptomatology and plasma levels. As a model we chose intoxications with Vesparax®, a very potent hypnotic drug. Vesparax® is a combination of 150 mg secobarbital, 50 mg brallobarbital and 50 mg hydroxyzine per tablet. We made this choice because intoxications with this drug occur frequently in the Netherlands and because they are often fatal (van Heijst et al. 1976). From the first results of this study it is evident that for an evaluation of the efficiency of haemoperfusion, it is not sufficient to determine the pre- and post-perfusion plasma levels (de Groot et al. 1977). The plasma levels generally did not change at all while the clearances were considerable (table 1). This shows clearly why negative criticism is so often heard about the results obtained in haemoperfusion. It is generally expected to find a distinct decline of the plasma level. Clearance values often are not determined because it takes time, is expensive and the results are not immediately known. Often there exists no correlation between the clinical symptoms and the plasma levels. During haemoperfusion the completely absent reflexes returned rapidly to normal and in some cases the patient regains consciousness.

To be sure that haemoperfusion or haemodialysis will achieve the desired result it is necessary to know the plasma levels before the start of these procedures. As a result of this condition in our department many haemoperfusions requested on clinical grounds had to be cancelled. In the Department of Reanimation and Clinical Toxicology, 800–900 patients are admitted every year and about 300–400 of these are intoxicated. The routine toxicological analysis of these patients is performed as a 24-hour service in the toxicological laboratory of the University Hospital Pharmacy

Table 1. Plasma levels, clearance values and quantities of brallobarbital and secobarbital removed by haemoperfusion therapy in seven cases of Vesparax® intoxication.

Case drug no.	Pre-perfusion plasma level (mg/l)	Post-perfusion plasma level (mg/l)	Clearance after ½ h (ml/min)	Clearance after 3 h (ml/min)	Amount removed (g)
1. Brallobarbital	48	41	120	57	0.54
Secobarbital	27	28	86	78	0.42
2. Brallobarbital	106	67	163	88	2.13
Secobarbital	41	42	160	67	0.88
3. Brallobarbital	26	22	99	58	0.30
Secobarbital	9	9	95	65	0.17
4. Brallobarbital	40	26	46	67	0.42
Secobarbital	33	20	58	74	0.36
5. Brallobarbital	32	29	31	14	0.13
Secobarbital	21	19	35	18	0.11
6. Brallobarbital	31	27	89	102	0.49
Secobarbital	22	21	97	96	0.39
7. Brallobarbital	8	5	115	56	0.07
Secobarbital	6	4	134	31	0.07

(J. Glerum, Pharm. D). Before a toxicological analysis is made the pharmacist inspects the patient and obtains all necessary information from the clinician on duty. As a result of this procedure the number of toxicological analyses is limited, but they are more adequately performed. For instance, the pharmacist will have detailed information on the drugs regularly taken by the patient, which may interfere with the analysis. The indication to perform a haemodialysis or haemoperfusion is also taken in consultation with the pharmacist. To give some idea of the kind and number of the qualitative and quantitative analyses considered necessary for the patients in our department a survey over 1977 is shown (table 2), to be discussed for its implications for treatment.

BARBITURATES

Intoxications with these drugs are frequent in the Netherlands, and have a high mortality rate. In total 117 analyses were done; the differentiation in the barbiturates is shown in table 2. From our own experience we composed a list of plasma levels of various barbiturates for which, in our opinion, intensive therapy is necessary (table 3).

NON-BARBITURATES

Non-barbiturates intoxications are less frequent. In the beginning we feared intoxications with methaqualone, about which we were warned by

Table 2. Number of quantitative analyses in plasma in Utrecht University Hospital in the course of 1977.

Barbiturates		Psychotropic drugs	
butobarbital	30	meprobamate	12
phenobarbital	30	amitriptyline	6
secobarbital	20	diazepam + N-desmethyldiazepam	9
vinylbital	10	chlordiazepoxide	1
cyclobarbital	6		
hexobarbital	6	Analgesic drugs	
pentobarbital	6	paracetamol	32
barbital	5	salicylates	30
amobarbital	2	oxyphenbutazone	1
butalbital	1		
methylphenobarbital	1	Miscellaneous drugs	
		alcohol	49
Non-barbiturate hypnotics		phenytoin	16
methaqualone	23	orphenadrine	2
trichloroethanol	13	theophylline	1
glutethimide	8	free bromide	1

Table 3. Plasma concentrations (mg/l) of some hypnotics above which intensive therapy is indicated.

Barbiturates	
phenobarbital	150–200
barbital	150–200
butobarbital	60–80
cyclobarbital	60
hexobarbital	30–40
pentobarbital	30–40
secobarbital	30–40
vinylbital	30–40
Non-barbiturates	
glutethimide	40–50
meprobamate	200

our Scottish colleagues (Lawson and Brown 1967) but in our experience the prognosis is not unfavourable.

We are more and more confronted with intoxications with chloralhydrate, a drug which is considered safer than the modern hypnotic drugs because it is often prescribed for youngsters and elderly people. However, taken in an overdose, it appears to be cardiotoxic. We are interested in the plasma level of trichloroethanol, one of the principal metabolites, to obtain some insight into the gravity of the intoxication (van Heijst et al. 1977).

Glutethimide intoxications are rare but have many complications, especially in the lungs. If the plasma level is higher than 40–50 mg/1, haemoperfusion must seriously be considered.

PSYCHOTROPIC DRUGS

Meprobamate intoxications are notorious for hypotension. In cases with plasma levels higher than 200 mg/1 haemoperfusion is indicated. In intoxications with tricyclic antidepressants the determination of plasma level is not useful for therapy because of the very large volume of distribution of these drugs, and thence the low plasma-to-tissue concentration ratio. Although intoxications with benzodiazepines (diazepam) appear to be not very serious we saw a long-lasting coma after we discontinued prolonged administrations of high doses in a patient with tetanus. The plasma level of diazepam falls quickly, but the metabolite N-desmethyldiazepam level remains high for a long period. In the differentiation of the origin of the comatose state of the patient these findings can be important.

ANALGESIC DRUGS

Intoxications with these drugs are not a serious problem in the Netherlands
as contrasted with Britain. But if unfortunately paracetamol replaces phena-
cetin in the near future, regrettable accidents will follow. In Great Britain
in 1975, 105 patients died from paracetamol poisoning alone while in another 121 deaths paracetamol was involved in combination with other drugs.
If the patient with a serious paracetamol intoxication is not treated within
ten hours he will die as a result of liver necrosis. As most of the patients
arrive in the hospital later than ten hours after ingestion the prognosis in
severe intoxications is poor. The determination of the plasma level is very

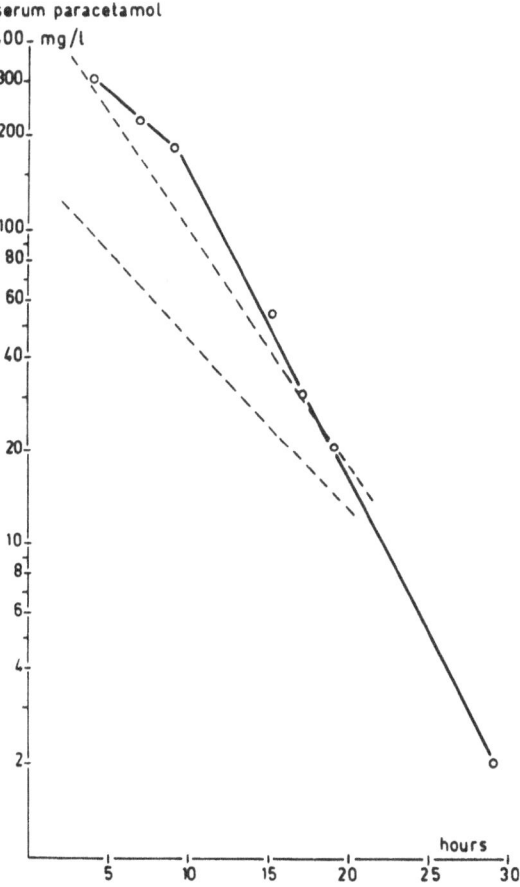

Figure 3. Course of paracetamol serum levels in a patient with a severe paracetamol
intoxication.

important: when plotted against time after ingestion of the drug, a good impression of the severity of the intoxication is obtained.

Fig. 3 shows the course of the serum levels in a patient with a severe intoxication treated with acetylcysteine orally. The patient recovered while no disturbances in liver functions tests were observed. According to James et al. (1975) nine out of eleven patients with plasma levels above the upper dotted line indicated in fig. 3 had severe liver biopsy changes while only two of seventeen patients whose plasma paracetamol levels lay below the lower dotted line showed mild biopsy changes.

In cases of salicylate intoxication, the determination of plasma levels is essential. In the nomogram of Done (1960) the expected severity of the intoxication at varying time intervals after ingestion can be estimated (fig. 4). In severe intoxications haemodialysis or haemoperfusion is indicated.

MISCELLANEOUS DRUGS

Because the combination of drugs with alcohol is often used in intentional intoxications, and their action thus intensified, it is recommended that the ethanol plasma level be determined. In an intoxication of ethanol alone haemodialysis is indicated if the plasma level is 4–5 g/l, but especially with alcohol the clinical state of the patient must certainly be taken into con-

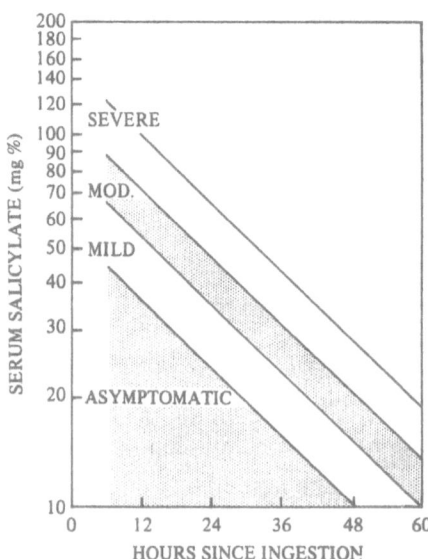

Figure 4. Nomogram of Done (1960) for the evaluation of salicylate intoxications.

sideration. In a chronic alcoholic the plasma level may be 6 g/l without the patient being in coma.

Intoxications with phenytoin in combination with phenobarbital occur quite frequently. In fig. 5, the course of plasma levels of such a combined intoxication during haemoperfusion in a 42-year old male is demonstrated. Some rebound was observed for phenobarbital, but more so for phenytoin, resulting in increasing plasma levels. Five hours after haemoperfusion the

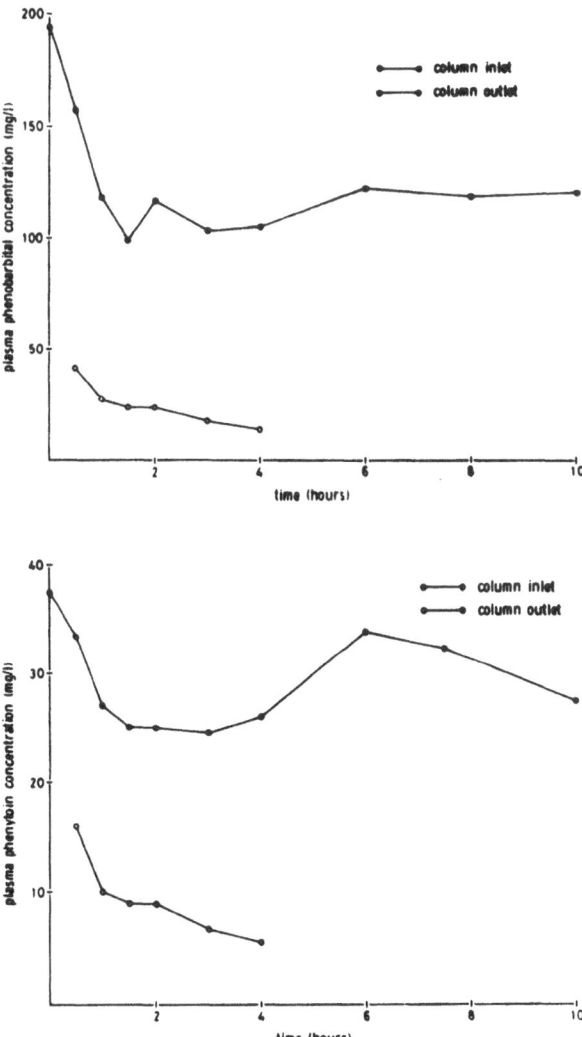

Figure 5. Course of phenobarbital and phenytoin plasma levels in a patient with a combined intoxication, who was treated with haemoperfusion. Samples were taken before and after the haemoperfusion column.

Table 4. Minimum needs for toxicological analysis of drugs.

Qualitative and quantitative in plasma	Qualitative in urine or stomach contents
barbiturates	benzodiazepines
phenytoin	phenothiazines
glutethimide	tricyclic antidepressants
lithium	quinine
meprobamate	codeine
paracetamol	amphetamine
carbromal	cocaine
salicylates	morphine
methaqualone	pethidine
diazepam + N-desmethyldiazepam	methadone
dextropropoxyphene	dextromoramide
trichloroethanol	

reflexes, initially totally absent, were normal again while the blood levels were still high.

In hospitals where severely intoxicated patients are frequently admitted, the minimum needs for toxicological analysis of drugs, qualitative as well as quantitative, are mentioned in table 4.

The result of these analyses is of primary interest in well equipped hospitals because they have immediate consequences for intensive treatment. In this table the drugs are also mentioned for which only qualitative analysis gives sufficient information and quantitative analysis is not relevant for the treatment.

REFERENCES

Done, A.K., Salicylate intoxication. *Pediatrics* 26, 800 (1960).
De Groot, G., Maes, R.A.A. and van Heijst, A.N.P., The use of haemoperfusion in the elimination of absorbed drug mixtures in acute intoxications. *Neth. J. Med.* 20, 142 (1977).
Van Heijst, A.N.P., Douze, J.M.C. and Pikaar, S.A., National Vergiftigingen Informatie Centrum *Ned. T. Geneesk.* 120, 206 (1976).
Van Heijst, A.N.P., Zimmerman, A.N.E. and Pikaar, S.A., Chloralhydraat: het vergeten vergif. *Ned. T. Geneesk.* 121, 1537–1539 (1977).
James, O., Lesna, M., Roberts, S.H., Pulman, L., Douglas, A.P., Smith, P.A., and Watson A.J., Liver damage after paracetamol overdose: comparison of liver function tests, fasting serum bile acids and liver histology. *Lancet* 7935, 579 (1975).
Lawson, A.A.H. and Brown, S.S., Acute methaqualone (Mandrax) poisoning. *Scott. Med. J.* 12, 63 (1976).

18. EPILOGUE: AN ANIMAL PHARMACOLOGIST'S REFLECTIONS ON DRUG ASSAYS IN MAN

E.L. NOACH

The optimistic expectations of recent years that increasing use of drug assays in clinical practice would rapidly change physicians' attitudes in prescribing drugs have as yet not become true: with the extension of knowledge and experience more problems emerged than had been anticipated. Two factors are mainly responsible for the still rather wide gap between animal pharmacology (including pharmacokinetics) and parallel developments in drug studies in man: first, the large differences of human populations in genetic, alimentary, environmental and other background conditions introduce an unfavourable heterogeneity if compared to the stringent requirements of homogeneity in test animal colonies. Second, the impact of illness of varying degree on pharmacodynamic and pharmacokinetic processes in man as compared to high standards of animal health under laboratory conditions complicate the interpretation of many experimental results in clinical pharmacology.

Not among the least of the merits of the present symposium is the fact that, in addition to reports on many successful studies, the authors did not hesitate to mention numerous still unsolved problems in most fields of drug assay. By doing so, a solid motivation is given for directed efforts in search of achieving the ultimate goal of drug assays, namely to serve as a widely used, often indispensable help for the initiation and adjustment of pharmacotherapy, tailored to the needs of the individual patient.

In the following sections emphasis will be laid on those aspects which specially deserve further development; thus, this review mostly contains preview aspects of preceding contributions to this volume. However, it should be understood that views and recommendations expressed here are this author's opinions, which need not be shared by the authors from whose contributions they were derived.

PURPOSES OF DRUG ASSAYS

The most unambiguous purpose is the chemical diagnosis of drug intoxication. Whereas massive overdosage may be detected without too many difficulties (especially since in many cases anamnestic data are available), problems may arise if drug toxicity is enhanced by interactions with other drugs (e.g., digitalis intoxication during concomitant thiazide administration). In such cases, chemical analysis is of only limited value if not supplemented by clinical data. This underlines the urgent need for exchange of information between drug laboratory chemists and clinicians. Also, for cases of presumed but hitherto unknown interactional toxicity, facilities should be available for rapid initiation of model experiments in animals. Therefore, drug laboratories should have cordial connections with departments of (animal) pharmacology to secure adequate experimental support.

WHAT SHOULD BE MEASURED?

Extent and limitations
No simple rule of thumb is available as to the products to be assayed: should analytical efforts mainly be directed to the pharmacologically relevant substances administered, or should active metabolites be assayed too? Sometimes, as in the case of the antidepressant amitriptyline, the active metabolite (nortriptyline) could be determined also in view of its different kinetic properties: the therapeutic effect is dependent on the combined activity of both compounds. In other cases, such as bioassays of antibiotics, the method used does not discriminate between the mother substance and its active metabolites, since the latter also have an antibiotic action on the test bacteria. A possible complication in the interpretation of test results could then be that the patient's pathogenic bacteria may have a different sensitivity for such metabolites.

The exclusive measurement of *in*active metabolites has not been mentioned in the symposium. However, in cases where technical difficulties preclude determinations of the administered substance itself, the plasma metabolite level might serve as a useful parameter for drug absorption.

Material for analysis
In general, drug levels are determined in easily accessible material such as blood and its constituents, or urine, saliva, and so on. A more thorough exploration of other material for drug assays, closer to the site of action, would be worthwhile. In recent work in this laboratory, it was shown that suction blisters of the skin contain liquid which is probably identical to extracellular fluid, otherwise difficult to obtain (M.J. Herfst and H. van Rees, personal communication).

Sampling
In view of the importance of time-concentration relations in drug assays, intensive contacts between clinicians and laboratory workers are indispensable: the latter should not restrict their activities to analytical work but should also advise clinicians on optimal sampling procedures. Whereas such contacts can easily be established in large hospitals having their own

drug laboratories, complications may arise when centralized laboratories extend their services to peripheral hospitals and individual medical practitioners. A thorough knowledge of pharmacokinetics then should be the common basis for mutual understanding. Fortunately, both in medical and pharmaceutical teaching curricula, increasing attention is given to this branch of pharmacology. This tendency should be encouraged.

Selection of drugs
The extent of monitoring drug levels depends on several factors. Foremost among them are technical possibilities and facilities; perhaps even more important are expectations concerning the correlation between dosage and blood level: the more unpredictable this correlation is, the more urgent is the need for assistance of a drug laboratory. In addition, drug assays serve the purpose of checking on patient compliance in regularly taking the prescribed drugs.

In present conditions, repeated drug assays are indispensable for anti-epileptics, antidepressants, lithium, some antibiotics and some cytostatics. As to these drugs, there are large inter-individual differences in absorption, metabolic fate and excretion, so that uniform dosage schedules are of no use. Furthermore, owing to enzyme induction and similar factors, even under a constant dosage scheme gradual shifts in equilibrium drug levels may occur in one and the same patient. Finally, especially in chronic therapy, the course of the disease may influence the fate and hence the level of the drugs used.

In the Netherlands, excellent results of therapy with oral anticoagulants could be obtained thanks to a nationwide system by which nearly all patients are regularly monitored. This shows the advantages and possibilities of such monitoring procedures (in this example, not drug *levels* but drug *effects* are assayed). With other classes of drugs such as digitalis glycosides and beta-blockers, regular drug assays, if not indispensable, are nevertheless important, especially in order to prevent overdosages. Of course, drug assays and pharmacokinetic studies should be performed with many drugs, especially those which have high threshold concentrations and those with narrow safety margins. From such studies, rules and priorities concerning clinical drug assays may emerge, although it may be expected that a continuous evolution in opinions on relevance, therapeutic consequences and exigencies of laboratory facilities will occur.

TECHNICAL PROVISIONS

In most hospitals there will nearly always be a gap between technical possibilities as provided by scientific developments and the possibilities of obtaining adequate equipment: whereas with sophisticated and mostly expensive apparatus and a generous qualitative and quantitative input of manpower hardly any drug will escape detection in biological material, most laboratories will be somewhat limited in their equipment. In view of the necessity of close contacts between clinicians and laboratory workers, decentralization of drug assay facilities is desirable. This requires the use of simple, reliable and uniform analytical procedures. At present, radio-immunoassays in their several modifications seem to fulfil such an approach optimally. Furthermore, the establishment of inter-laboratory comparison of analytical results (as already exists for anticonvulsant drugs) should be encouraged.

RELEVANCE OF DRUG LEVELS

Limitations in this field are all too obvious. Unless much more is known about the causes underlying discrepancies and uncertainties, it may be difficult to convince some hospital managements about the necessity of establishing drug assay facilities.

Relations between dose and drug levels
With many drugs, there are large inter-individual differences in the relation between administered dose and the ensuing time-concentration curve. Among these are oral anticoagulants, anticonvulsants, antidepressants, beta-blockers, lidocaine, lithium and many others. Much work has to be done in order to obtain an insight into the factors determining such differences. Also, simple routine tests should be developed in order to predict in individual patients absorptive and drug-metabolizing capacities. However, one should be aware of the hazards of treating a patient's drug level rather than his illness. In drugs with a relatively rapid effect, such as antibiotics, antiarrhythmics, some hypotensives, it is not too difficult to adjust dosage schedules with reference to drug effects and drug levels. However, in drugs with prolonged latent periods such as tricyclic anti-depressants, methodology has to be improved in order to establish optimal dosage schedules as soon as possible after the initiation of therapy.

Relations between blood levels and pharmacodynamic effects
A disappointingly small amount of hard facts is available about these relations in man. In view of the frequent poor correlation between dosage and blood level, as discussed in the previous paragraph, this means that dose-effect relations are even more unpredictable. This unsatisfactory situation may be mainly due to the heterogeneity of patient populations, as was mentioned in the introductory paragraph of this paper. In addition, parameters for assessment of drug effects in man are in many instances

notoriously insufficient. For instance, the *prevention* of certain symptoms (such as epileptic seizures, or insomnia, or vertigo) is a poor yardstick for evaluation of dose- or concentration-effect relations. Furthermore, a most important factor often seems to have been overlooked, namely the impact of disease on the extent and efficacy of drug effects. The degree of illness may interact with drug effects, for instance by causing a shift in the dose-effect curve. Such shifts could contribute to the large inter-individual variability in drug effects. Admittedly, methods of quantification of disease symptoms are only available in a few cases; therefore, much attention should be given to further development of methodology in this particular field. Finally, in most discussions on the therapeutic relevance of drug assays, the natural history of the disease to be treated is very rarely taken into consideration: perhaps too much confidence is put in the expectation that a solid double-blind experimental design will circumvent problems in this field.

AN EPILOGUE'S EPILOGUE: SOME PERSONAL RECOMMENDATIONS

Clinical pharmacologists and clinicians should intensify efforts to quantify symptoms of disease and improve the assessment of pharmacological effects in man. This should be done under the auspices of an international authority such as the World Health Organization in order to prevent the simultaneous emergence of multiple and mutually incomparable classification systems. Furthermore, work along these lines should be performed in close co-operation with experts in the field of drug assays and clinical pharmacokinetics. Such a multidisciplinary approach could be optimally pursued in institutes for clinical pharmacology with access to large numbers of patients and intensive contacts with research centres for animal pharmacology, medicinal chemistry (including pharmaceutical industries) and pharmaceutical technology. Not only older and newer active substances should be investigated, but also comparative studies should be done on different formulations of the same drug. In this way independent laboratories could contribute to quality control of related commercial preparations and hence could help to establish a more rational pharmacotherapy.

INDEX